T0263338

Gastroesophageal Reflux Disease

Editor

JOEL E. RICHTER

GASTROENTEROLOGY CLINICS OF NORTH AMERICA

www.gastro.theclinics.com

Consulting Editor
GARY W. FALK

March 2014 • Volume 43 • Number 1

ELSEVIER

1600 John F. Kennedy Boulevard • Suite 1800 • Philadelphia, Pennsylvania, 19103-2899

http://www.theclinics.com

GASTROENTEROLOGY CLINICS OF NORTH AMERICA Volume 43, Number 1
March 2014 ISSN 0889-8553, ISBN-13: 978-0-323-29028-9

Editor: Kerry Holland
Developmental Editor: Susan Showalter

© 2014 Elsevier Inc. All rights reserved.

This periodical and the individual contributions contained in it are protected under copyright by Elsevier, and the following terms and conditions apply to their use:

Photocopying

Single photocopies of single articles may be made for personal use as allowed by national copyright laws. Permission of the Publisher and payment of a fee is required for all other photocopying, including multiple or systematic copying, copying for advertising or promotional purposes, resale, and all forms of document delivery. Special rates are available for educational institutions that wish to make photocopies for non-profit educational classroom use. For information on how to seek permission visit www.elsevier.com/permissions or call: (+44) 1865 843830 (UK)/ (+1) 215 239 3804 (USA).

Derivative Works

Subscribers may reproduce tables of contents or prepare lists of articles including abstracts for internal circulation within their institutions. Permission of the Publisher is required for resale or distribution outside the institution. Permission of the Publisher is required for all other derivative works, including compilations and translations (please consult www.elsevier.com/permissions).

Electronic Storage or Usage

Permission of the Publisher is required to store or use electronically any material contained in this periodical, including any article or part of an article (please consult www.elsevier.com/permissions). Except as outlined above, no part of this publication may be reproduced, stored in a retrieval system or transmitted in any form or by any means, electronic, mechanical, photocopying, recording or otherwise, without prior written permission of the Publisher.

Notice

No responsibility is assumed by the Publisher for any injury and/or damage to persons or property as a matter of products liability, negligence or otherwise, or from any use or operation of any methods, products, instructions or ideas contained in the material herein. Because of rapid advances in the medical sciences, in particular, independent verification of diagnoses and drug dosages should be made. Although all advertising material is expected to conform to ethical (medical) standards, inclusion in this publication does not constitute a guarantee or endorsement of the quality or value of such product or of the claims made of it by its manufacturer.

Gastroenterology Clinics of North America (ISSN 0889-8553) is published quarterly by Elsevier Inc., 360 Park Avenue South, New York, NY 10010-1710. Months of issue are March, June, September, and December. Business and Editorial Offices: 1600 John F. Kennedy Blvd., Suite 1800, Philadelphia, PA 19103-2899. Customer Service Office: 6277 Sea Harbor Drive, Orlando, FL 32887-4800. Periodicals postage paid at New York, NY and additional mailing offices. Subscription prices are $320.00 per year (US individuals), $160.00 per year (US students), $530.00 per year (US institutions), $350.00 per year (Canadian individuals), $651.00 per year (Canadian institutions), $445.00 per year (international individuals), $220.00 per year (international students), and $651.00 per year (international institutions). Foreign air speed delivery is included in all *Clinics* subscription prices. All prices are subject to change without notice. **POSTMASTER**: Send address changes to *Gastroenterology Clinics of North America*, Elsevier Health Sciences Division, Subscription Customer Service, 3251 Riverport Lane, Maryland Heights, MO 63043. Telephone: 1-800-654-2452 (U.S. and Canada); 314-447-8871 (outside U.S. and Canada). Fax: 314-447-8029. E-mail: journalscustomerservice-usa@elsevier.com (for print support); journalsonlinesupport-usa@elsevier.com (for online support).

Reprints. For copies of 100 or more, of articles in this publication, please contact the Commercial Reprints Department, Elsevier Inc., 360 Part Avenue South, New York, New York 10010-1710. Tel. 212-633-3874, Fax: 212-633-3820, E-mail: reprints@elsevier.com.

Gastroenterology Clinics of North America is also published in Italian by Il Pensiero Scientifico Editore, Rome, Italy; and in Portuguese by Interlivros Edicoes Ltda., Rua Commandante Coelho 1085, 21250 Cordovil, Rio de Janeiro, Brazil.

Gastroenterology Clinics of North America is covered in *MEDLINE/PubMed (Index Medicus), Excerpta Medica, Current Contents/Clinical Medicine, Science Citation Index, ISI/BIOMED*, and *BIOSIS*.

Printed and bound by CPI Group (UK) Ltd, Croydon, CR0 4YY

Contributors

CONSULTING EDITOR

GARY W. FALK, MD, MS
Professor of Medicine, Division of Gastroenterology, University of Pennsylvania Perelman School of Medicine, Philadelphia, Pennsylvania

EDITOR

JOEL E. RICHTER, MD, FACP, MACG
Professor of Medicine, Hugh F. Culverhouse Chair for Esophageal Disorders, Director, Division of Digestive Diseases and Nutrition, Director, Joy McCann Culverhouse, Center for Esophageal and Swallowing Disorders, University of South Florida Morsani College of Medicine, Tampa, Florida

AUTHORS

SAMI R. ACHEM, MD, FACG, FACP
Professor, Department of Medicine, Mayo Clinic College of Medicine, Jacksonville, Florida

MARK E. BAKER, MD, FARS, FSCBT/MR
Professor of Radiology, Cleveland Clinic Lerner College of Medicine, Case Western Reserve University; Staff Radiologist, Abdominal Imaging, Imaging Institute; Digestive Disease Institute and Cancer Institute, Cleveland Clinic, Cleveland, Ohio

GUY E. BOECKXSTAENS, MD, PhD
Department of Gastroenterology, Translational Research Center for Gastrointestinal Disorders (TARGID), University Hospital of Leuven, University of Leuven, Leuven, Belgium

DUSTIN A. CARLSON, MD
Department of Medicine, Feinberg School of Medicine, Northwestern University, Chicago, Illinois

PAUL CHANG, MD
Professor of Medicine, Section of Gastroenterology, Temple University School of Medicine, Philadelphia, Pennsylvania

JOAN W. CHEN, MD
Clinical Lecturer, Division of Gastroenterology, University of Michigan Medical School, Ann Arbor, Michigan

KENNETH R. DEVAULT, MD, FACG, FACP
Professor, Department of Medicine, Mayo Clinic College of Medicine, Jacksonville, Florida

DAVID M. EINSTEIN, MD, FARS
Clinical Professor of Radiology, Cleveland Clinic Lerner College of Medicine, Case Western Reserve University; Vice-Chairman, Education, and Staff Radiologist, Abdominal Imaging, Imaging Institute, Cleveland Clinic, Cleveland, Ohio

DAVID S. ESTORES, MD
Assistant Professor of Clinical Medicine, Division of Gastroenterology, Hepatology and Nutrition, University of Florida, Gainesville, Florida

FRANK FRIEDENBERG, MD, MS (Epi)
Senior Fellow, Section of Gastroenterology, Temple University School of Medicine, Philadelphia, Pennsylvania

C. PRAKASH GYAWALI, MD
Professor of Medicine, Division of Gastroenterology, Washington University School of Medicine, St Louis, Missouri

DAVID KIM, MD
Resident, Division of General Surgery, University of South Florida, Tampa, Florida

RYAN D. MADANICK, MD
Assistant Professor of Medicine; Director, UNC Gastroenterology and Hepatology Fellowship Program; Vice-Chief for Education, Division of Gastroenterology and Hepatology, University of North Carolina School of Medicine, Chapel Hill, North Carolina

MICHAEL MELLO, MD
Division of Gastroenterology, Washington University School of Medicine, St Louis, Missouri

JOHN E. PANDOLFINO, MD, MSCI
Department of Medicine, Feinberg School of Medicine, Northwestern University, Chicago, Illinois

WOUT O. ROHOF, MD, PhD
Department of Gastroenterology and Hepatology, Academic Medical Center, Amsterdam, The Netherlands

JOEL H. RUBENSTEIN, MD, MSc
Research Scientist, Veterans Affairs Center for Clinical Management Research; Assistant Professor, Division of Gastroenterology, University of Michigan Medical School, Ann Arbor, Michigan

VIRENDER K. SHARMA, MD, FACG, AGAF, FASGE
Director, Arizona Digestive Health, Gilbert, Arizona

MARCELO F. VELA, MD, MSCR, FACG
Associate Professor of Medicine, Director of GI Motility, Division of Gastroenterology and Hepatology, Michael E. DeBakey VA Medical Center, Baylor College of Medicine, Houston, Texas

VIC VELANOVICH, MD
Professor, Division of General Surgery, University of South Florida, Tampa, Florida

Contents

> The prevalence of gastroesophageal reflux disease (GERD) symptoms increased approximately 50% until the mid-1990s, when it plateaued. The incidence of complications related to GERD including hospitalization, esophageal strictures, esophageal adenocarcinoma, and mortality also increased during that time period, but the increase in esophageal adenocarcinoma has since slowed, and the incidence of strictures has decreased since the mid-1990s. GERD is responsible for the greatest direct costs in the United States of any gastrointestinal disease, and most of those expenditures are for pharmacotherapy. Risk factors for GERD include obesity, poor diet, lack of physical activity, consumption of tobacco and alcohol, and respiratory diseases.

> Gastroesophageal reflux disease (GERD) is one of the most common digestive diseases in the Western world, with typical symptoms, such as heartburn, regurgitation, or retrosternal pain, reported by 15% to 20% of the general population. The pathophysiology of GERD is multifactorial. Our understanding of these factors has significantly improved in recent years, with increased understanding of the acid pocket and hiatal hernia and how these factors interact. Although our insight has significantly increased over the past years, more studies are required to better understand symptom generation in GERD, especially in patients with therapy-resistant symptoms.

> There are problems with the definition, assessment, and measurement of gastroesophageal reflux disease (GERD). The Reflux Disease Questionnaire and the GERD questionnaire are patient-reported outcome (PRO) measures for use in a primary care setting, which are easy to use and are validated. There is no widely accepted definition of a proton pump inhibitor test and performance of the test in the clinical setting is not standardized. The use of the PRO measures in primary care with predetermined cutoff

values may help to reduce the cost of diagnosing GERD and increasing rates of response for evaluated patients to acid suppression.

Endoscopy is commonly performed for the diagnosis and management of gastroesophageal reflux disease (GERD). Endoscopy allows the physician to evaluate esophageal mucosa for evidence of esophagitis and Barrett esophagus, to obtain mucosal biopsies for evaluation of such conditions as eosinophilic esophagitis and diagnosis and grading of Barrett esophagus, and to apply various therapies. In a patient with suboptimal response to GERD therapy, endoscopy excludes other etiologies as a cause of patients' symptoms. Newer endoscopic therapies for GERD are available or are in development. Advances in imaging techniques in development will improve the diagnostic yield of endoscopy and may replace the need for mucosal biopsies.

The barium esophagram is an integral part of the assessment and management of patients with gastroesophageal reflux disease (GERD) before, and especially after, antireflux procedures. While many of the findings on the examination can be identified with endosocopy, a gastric emptying study and an esophageal motility examination, the barium esophagram is better at demonstrating the anatomic findings after antireflux surgery, especially in symptomatic patients. These complementary examinations, when taken as a whole, fully evaluate a patient with suspected GERD as well as symptomatic patients after antireflux procedures.

High-resolution manometry (HRM) allows nuanced evaluation of esophageal motor function, and more accurate evaluation of lower esophageal sphincter (LES) function, in comparison with conventional manometry. Pathophysiologic correlates of gastroesophageal reflux disease (GERD) and esophageal peristaltic performance are well addressed by this technique. HRM may alter the surgical decision by assessment of esophageal peristaltic function and exclusion of esophageal outflow obstruction before antireflux surgery. Provocative testing during HRM may assess esophageal smooth muscle peristaltic reserve and help predict the likelihood of transit symptoms following antireflux surgery. HRM represents a continuously evolving new technology that compliments the evaluation and management of GERD.

Detection of acid and nonacid reflux using esophageal reflux monitoring, which includes conventional and wireless pH monitoring and pH impedance, can be a valuable diagnostic tool when used appropriately in the assessment of patients with gastroesophageal reflux disease. Reflux monitoring may be especially helpful if a management change is desired, such as when initial or empirical treatment is ineffective. However, each of these methods has its limitations, which need to be accounted for in their clinical use. Indications, test performance, interpretation, and clinical applications of esophageal reflux monitoring, as well as their limitations, are discussed in this review.

This article reviews the evaluation and management of patients with suspected extraesophageal manifestations of gastroesophageal reflux disease, such as asthma, chronic cough, and laryngitis, which are commonly encountered in gastroenterology practices. Otolaryngologists and gastroenterologists commonly disagree upon the underlying cause for complaints in patients with one of the suspected extraesophageal reflux syndromes. The accuracy of diagnostic tests (laryngoscopy, endoscopy, and pH- or pH-impedance monitoring) for patients with suspected extraesophageal manifestations of gastroesophageal reflux disease is suboptimal. An empiric trial of proton pump inhibitors in patients without alarm features can help some patients, but the response to therapy is variable.

The mainstay of pharmacological therapy for gastroesophageal reflux disease (GERD) is gastric acid suppression with proton pump inhibitors (PPIs), which are superior to histamine-2 receptor antagonists for healing erosive esophagitis and achieving symptomatic relief. However, up to one-third of patients may not respond to PPI therapy, creating the need for alternative treatments. Potential approaches include transient lower esophageal sphincter relaxation inhibitors, augmentation esophageal defense mechanisms by improving esophageal clearance or enhancing epithelial repair, and modulation of sensory pathways responsible for GERD symptoms. This review discusses the effectiveness of acid suppression and the data on alternative pharmacological approaches for the treatment of GERD.

Surgical management of gastroesophageal reflux disease has evolved from relatively invasive procedures requiring open laparotomy or thoracotomy to minimally invasive laparoscopic techniques. Although side effects may still occur, with careful patient selection and good technique, the overall symptomatic control leads to satisfaction rates in the 90% range. Unfortunately, the next evolution to endoluminal techniques has not been as successful. Reliable devices are still awaited that consistently produce long-term symptomatic relief with correction of pathologic reflux. However, newer laparoscopically placed devices hold promise in achieving equivalent symptomatic relief with fewer side effects. Clinical trials are still forthcoming.

Sami R. Achem and Kenneth R. DeVault

Gastroesophageal reflux disease is a common disorder in all patients but a particular problem in the elderly, for whom the disease often presents with advanced mucosal damage and other complications. Symptoms are also not as reliable an indication of disease severity in older patients. Likewise, therapy is more difficult because of potential side effects and drug interactions.

Paul Chang and Frank Friedenberg

Epidemiologic data have demonstrated that obesity is an important risk factor for the development of gastroesophageal reflux disease (GERD). There is also accumulating data that obesity is associated with complications related to longstanding reflux such as erosive esophagitis, Barrett esophagus, and esophageal adenocarcinoma. Central obesity, rather than body mass index, appears to be more closely associated with these complications. Surgical data are confounded by the concomitant repair of prevalent hiatal hernias in many patients.

GASTROENTEROLOGY
CLINICS OF NORTH AMERICA

DOWNLOAD Free App!

Review Articles
THE CLINICS

NOW AVAILABLE FOR YOUR iPhone and iPad

Foreword

Gastroesophageal Reflux Disease

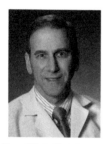

Gary W. Falk, MD, MS
Consulting Editor

Gastroesophageal reflux disease (GERD) remains one of the most common problems encountered in gastrointestinal clinical practice with over 8 million patient visits in the United States in 2009. Our understanding of the pathophysiology of this disorder has evolved considerably over the years, and the development of proton pump inhibitors almost twenty years ago radically altered both the diagnostic and the therapeutic approach to GERD. The effectiveness of this class of drugs led us to believe that we had this disease solved. However, in ensuing years it has become clear that the problem of GERD remains and the spectrum of the disease has changed to more challenging presentations, such as refractory GERD and a myriad of proposed extraesophageal manifestations. This has led to significant confusion regarding the optimal approach to these patients.

As such, the beginning of 2014 is an ideal time to address many of the evolving questions in clinical practice related to GERD, including

- What is the significance of the acid pocket?
- What is refractory GERD and what is the optimal diagnostic approach to these patients?
- What is a rational sequence for testing in patients where there is diagnostic uncertainty?
- Is nonacidic reflux really of any clinical significance?
- Is there any role for the new alternative endoscopic and surgical approaches now, given the prior limitations of endoscopic approaches to GERD?
- Are there any new medical therapies forthcoming?
- What are the implications of the obesity epidemic on the management of GERD?

To address these issues and more, Joel E. Richter, MD, one of the true giants in esophageal disease and my own valued mentor, has assembled established experts

Gastroenterol Clin N Am 43 (2014) xi–xii
http://dx.doi.org/10.1016/j.gtc.2014.01.001
0889-8553/14/$ – see front matter © 2014 Elsevier Inc. All rights reserved.

in the field to help us improve our understanding of GERD in the New Year. I think you will enjoy this issue of *Gastroenterology Clinics of North America*, which should enhance your approach to this common clinical problem.

Gary W. Falk, MD, MS
Division of Gastroenterology
University of Pennsylvania Perelman School of Medicine
9th Floor Penn Tower
1 Convention Avenue
Philadelphia, PA 19104-4311, USA

E-mail address:
Gary.Falk@uphs.upenn.edu

Preface

What's New in Gastroesophageal Reflux Disease for 2014

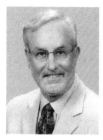

Joel E. Richter, MD, FACP, MACG
Editor

It is my pleasure to present you with this issue of *Gastroenterology Clinics of North America*. The issue focuses on a common disease—gastroesophageal reflux disease (GERD)—which is near and dear to me. My goals were two-fold: (1) to introduce the readership to some up and coming stars in esophageal diseases as well as some old friends, and (2) to give the clinical readership practical information generated over the last 5 years to help them manage GERD and its medical and surgical complications. I'm pleased with the outcomes and hope you are too.

The issue begins with an article on the epidemiology of GERD. Did you know the prevalence of GERD plateaued in the middle 1990s but it still incurs the highest annual direct costs of all digestive diseases in the United States? The next article has a European flavor, reviewing the pathophysiology of GERD with new information on the acid pocket and its interactions with sliding and fixed hiatal hernias.

The next five articles update the clinician on our diagnostic testing for GERD. These tests are of increasing importance as we understand the poor sensitivity of GERD symptoms and the unreliability of the proton pump test in the general community. Endoscopy will always be the first test for investigating GERD, but we are "seeing" so much more with narrow band imaging, high magnification endoscopy, and the newest technologies, confocal laser endomicroscopy and optical coherence tomography. However, don't forget the simple barium esophagram, which has a critical role in the preoperative assessment of the GERD patient and if postsurgical problems occur. High-resolution manometry can help us exclude esophageal outflow obstruction mimicking GERD and is fast becoming a preoperative test that can help alter surgical decisions. We have multiple available reflux tests, but there is confusion about which test to perform and whether to perform "on or off" proton pump inhibitors therapy. Furthermore, there has been much discussion about non-acid reflux, but is its

Gastroenterol Clin N Am 43 (2014) xiii–xiv
http://dx.doi.org/10.1016/j.gtc.2013.12.004
0889-8553/14/$ – see front matter © 2014 Elsevier Inc. All rights reserved.

identification alone in intractable patients' criteria for surgery or do we still need to define the presence of our old reliable friend—acid reflux?

The last four articles tackle treatments of GERD and extraesophageal GERD as well as specific issues in our elderly and/or obese patients. Did you know the Restech device is poorly validated in extraesophageal GERD and that many patients with chronic cough may have a sensory neuropathic cough potentially responding well to gabapentin? Why did the potassium-competitive acid blockers and GABA-B agonist–like medications fail in their clinical trials and is there anything new on the medical horizon? Surgical therapies have had their "ups and downs" but seem to be coming back with concerns about the long-term side effects of proton pump inhibitors. However, there are still worries about postop symptoms of dysphagia and gas bloat. Endoscopic surgical treatments are again appearing on the scene, but totally novel treatments like lower esophageal sphincter augmentation with magnetic beads and electrical stimulation of the lower esophageal sphincter may be the surgical wave of the future. Older patients have changes in their esophageal physiology that predispose them to more severe GERD and sometimes mask the severity of their disease. Finally, the obesity epidemic is a major contributing factor to the rise in GERD prevalence and all of its associated complications. Patients with reflux frequently undergo bariatric surgery and clinicians need to be aware that some of these operations can markedly worsen GERD.

I personally want to thank all the authors and coauthors for their excellent contributions to this edition of *Gastroenterology Clinics of North America*. I'm confident that you will find the information in these pages to be current, comprehensive, and highly clinically relevant.

Joel E. Richter, MD, FACP, MACG
Division of Digestive Diseases and Nutrition
Joy McCann Culverhouse
Center for Esophageal and Swallowing Disorders
University of South Florida Morsani College of Medicine
Tampa, FL 33612, USA

E-mail address:
jrichte1@health.usf.edu

Epidemiology of Gastroesophageal Reflux Disease

Joel H. Rubenstein, MD, MSc[a,b,*], Joan W. Chen, MD[b]

KEYWORDS

- Prevalence • Incidence • Risk factors • Esophageal strictures
- Esophageal neoplasms • Cost

KEY POINTS

- Frequent GERD symptoms are encountered in 20% of North Americans.
- The prevalence of GERD symptoms rose, and then plateaued in the mid-1990s.
- GERD incurs the highest annual direct costs of all digestive diseases in the United States.
- Pharmaceutical cost is responsible for most of the direct cost of GERD management.
- Risk factors for GERD include obesity, poor diet, lack of leisure physical activity, consumption of tobacco and alcohol, and respiratory disease.

INTRODUCTION

Gastroesophageal reflux disease (GERD) is a condition that develops when the reflux of gastric contents causes troublesome symptoms or complications.[1] GERD is responsible for some of the most common symptoms leading to presentation for medical care. The prevalence of GERD symptoms and the incidence of some of its complications have risen strikingly over the last few decades, leading to substantial economic impact. There are several potential explanations for these rising trends.

TRENDS IN THE PREVALENCE OF GERD AND INCIDENCE OF ITS COMPLICATIONS

Symptoms of GERD seem to be more common now than 25 years ago. In systematic reviews of population-based studies, El-Serag and colleagues[2,3] found that the prevalence of at least weekly symptoms of GERD rose approximately 50% until 1995, and that the prevalence has remained relatively constant since then (**Fig. 1**). The weighted-mean prevalence of at least weekly GERD symptoms is greatest in North America

[a] Veterans Affairs Center for Clinical Management Research, Ann Arbor, MI, USA; [b] Division of Gastroenterology, University of Michigan Medical School, Ann Arbor, MI, USA
* Corresponding author. VA Ann Arbor Healthcare System, 2215 Fuller Road, Mail Stop 111-D, Ann Arbor, MI 48105.
E-mail address: jhr@umich.edu

Gastroenterol Clin N Am 43 (2014) 1–14
http://dx.doi.org/10.1016/j.gtc.2013.11.006
0889-8553/14/$ – see front matter Published by Elsevier Inc.

gastro.theclinics.com

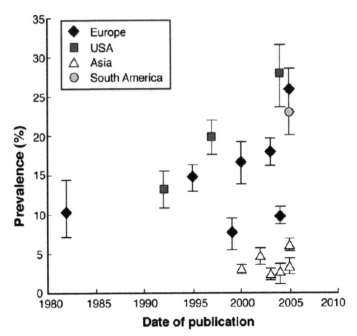

Fig. 1. Prevalence of at least weekly heartburn and/or acid regurgitation, or heartburn, with regard to the publication date of the 17 studies included in the Poisson regression analysis. Studies are categorized by geographic region (continent). (*From* El-Serag HB. Time trends of gastroesophageal reflux disease: a systematic review. Clin Gastroenterol Hepatol 2007;5:21; with permission.)

(19.8%), lowest in East Asia (5.2%), and intermediate in Europe and the Middle East (15.2% and 14.4%, respectively) (**Fig. 2**).[3] The rate of increase in the prevalence of symptoms seems to be similar across all geographic regions studied.[3]

The source studies for that systematic review were often limited because they did not account for the use of acid-reducing medications, which would be expected to mask GERD symptoms; because the use of such medications has increased, the true prevalence of GERD (including treated and untreated) may be greater than the estimates previously mentioned. In addition, the estimates were based primarily on studies of separate samples of populations obtained at different time points. One exception is the HUNT study, which administered surveys longitudinally to the same population over time; residents of a Norwegian county answered the questions between 1995 and 1997, and the same questions again between 2006 and 2009.[4] The prevalence of at least weekly GERD symptoms increased from 12% to 17% during that time period. GERD symptoms became more common in men and women, and in all age groups.

The incidence of complications of GERD also seems to have risen, but may have plateaued or even decreased since the mid-1990s. The proportion of hospitalizations in the US Veterans Affairs health care system with a primary or secondary discharge diagnosis of GERD increased fourfold between 1970 and 1996.[5] Mortality directly related to GERD is very rare, but analysis of US death certificates demonstrated an increase from 1 death per 1 million individuals per year to 2.1 per 1 million between 1979 and 1992.[5] In two community hospitals, the incidence of new esophageal strictures increased from 1986 to 1993, then decreased from 1994 to 2001, coinciding with

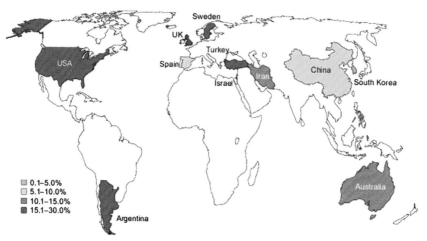

Fig. 2. Global distribution of the burden of gastroesophageal reflux disease. Sample-size weighted mean estimates of the prevalence of at least weekly heartburn and/or regurgitation in each country. (*From* El-Serag HB, Sweet S, Winchester CC, et al. Update on the epidemiology of gastro-oesophageal reflux disease: a systematic review. Gut 2013. http://dx.doi.org/10.1136/gutjnl-2012-304269; with permission.)

a large increase in prescriptions for proton pump inhibitors (PPIs).[6] In the US Veterans Affairs health care system, the incidence of new esophageal strictures decreased 12% as a proportion of all upper endoscopies from 1998 to 2003, and the 1-year incidence rate of recurrent strictures decreased 36%.[7] Similarly, within the US Medicare system, the proportion of upper endoscopies with a stricture declined 11% between 1992 and 2000, and the incidence of recurrent strictures decreased 30%, coinciding with the introduction of PPIs.[8]

The most feared complication of GERD is esophageal adenocarcinoma, a cancer that historically had been extremely rare. The cancer is fivefold as common in individuals with chronic GERD symptoms compared with those without GERD.[9] In 1991, a seminal study by Blot and colleagues[10] reported an alarming doubling of the incidence of esophageal adenocarcinoma from 1976 to 1987. The incidence of esophageal adenocarcinoma thereafter climbed to sevenfold the baseline incidence, and most recently occurs in the general US population in 2.6 per 100,000 patient-years.[11] World-wide, the incidence of esophageal adenocarcinoma has risen in most industrialized countries where there is a majority white population.[12,13] Despite the dramatic relative increase in the incidence of esophageal adenocarcinoma, it remains a rare disease in absolute terms. Indeed, even in men with chronic GERD symptoms, the incidence of colorectal cancer is likely threefold the incidence of esophageal adenocarcinoma, and women with GERD symptoms likely have an incidence of esophageal adenocarcinoma that is similar to the incidence of breast cancer in men.[14] Furthermore, the rising incidence may be reaching a plateau, because the increase in incidence has slowed in the United States since around 1997.[11,15] The plateauing of the incidence of esophageal adenocarcinoma might be in part related to the advent of PPIs.

Just as the incidence of esophageal adenocarcinoma has risen, there has been a dramatic rise in the incidence of diagnosed cases of Barrett's esophagus, the premalignant lesion associated with esophageal adenocarcinoma. For example, in a Dutch primary care database, the incidence of newly diagnosed cases of Barrett's esophagus rose from 11 per 100,000 patients in 1996 to 23 per 100,000 in 2003.[16] Similarly, in a large integrated US health care system, the incidence of diagnosed cases of Barrett's esophagus rose from 15 per 100,000 patient-years in 1998 to 24 per 100,000 in 2006.[17] In the same population, the prevalence of diagnosed Barrett's esophagus rose from less than 10 per 100,000 individuals in 1994 to 131 per 100,000 in 2006, with no sign of plateauing. These figures need to be interpreted with caution because estimating the changing incidence of Barrett's esophagus is more challenging than estimating the changing incidence of esophageal adenocarcinoma. Changes in the incidence of diagnosed Barrett's esophagus can be strongly influenced by changing patterns in the practice of upper endoscopy, both in terms of who gets referred for the procedure and which endoscopic and histologic findings are recognized as Barrett's esophagus. Hence, the proportion of individuals with Barrett's esophagus who are diagnosed with Barrett's esophagus has likely been increasing over the last few decades. Indeed, population-based studies of individuals invited to undergo upper endoscopy for research indicate that the true prevalence of Barrett's esophagus is much greater than suggested by the previously mentioned clinical studies, and at least 1300 per 100,000.[18,19] Therefore, it is unclear whether the incidence of Barrett's esophagus has truly been changing.

THE ECONOMIC IMPACT OF GERD

To assess the economic impact of GERD, one must consider direct and indirect costs. Direct health care costs include those incurred during office visits, diagnostic testing, treatment, and hospital admissions. Indirect costs include those from missed work because of symptoms or clinic visits, diminished productivity while at work, and impairment in performing daily activities.

Direct Health Care Costs

In a report using data from the late 1990s, GERD was found to be the digestive disease with the highest annual direct cost in the United States accounting for $9.3 billion.[20] A breakdown of the components of the direct cost is shown in **Fig. 3**. Pharmaceutical costs were responsible for most of the direct costs (63% or $5.9 billion). Hospital inpatient admissions ($2.5 billion), physician office visits ($603 million), hospital outpatient visits ($213 million), and hospital emergency visits ($78 million) made up the remainder

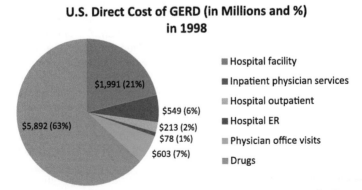

U.S. Direct Cost of GERD (in Millions and %) in 1998

$1,991 (21%)
$5,892 (63%)
$549 (6%)
$213 (2%)
$78 (1%)
$603 (7%)

■ Hospital facility
■ Inpatient physician services
■ Hospital outpatient
■ Hospital ER
■ Physician office visits
■ Drugs

Fig. 3. Components of direct costs of GERD (in millions and percentage). ER, emergency room. (*Data from* Sandler RS, Everhart JE, Donowitz M, et al. The burden of selected digestive diseases in the United States. Gastroenterology 2002;122:1500–11.)

of the cost.[20] In 2004, the direct costs of GERD were estimated to be even greater ($12.1 billion).[21]

Ambulatory care costs

When listed as a primary diagnosis, symptoms of GERD result in 4.6 million office encounters in the United States annually, and increases to 9.1 million visits annually if one includes visits in which a GERD diagnosis was listed as one of the top three diagnoses for the encounter.[20] Ambulatory care use in the United States for GERD has been up-trending in recent decades; between 1975 and 2004, the rate of ambulatory care visits with any diagnostic listing of GERD increased approximately 2000%.[21] GERD is the most frequently first-listed digestive system condition at ambulatory care visits, constituting 17.5% of all gastrointestinal diagnoses. Total ambulatory care costs, consisting of physician fees for office visits and any extra charges for procedures performed in offices, was estimated to be $1.4 billion in 2004.[21] This was the second highest contributor to total ambulatory care costs from digestive diseases.

Inpatient care costs

Gastroesophageal reflux (4.4 million) was the most common gastrointestinal discharge diagnosis among any listed diagnoses from hospital admissions based on an analysis of the 2009 US Nationwide Inpatient Sample of the Healthcare Cost and Utilization Project.[22] GERD was not commonly listed as the principal discharge diagnosis (13th digestive disease as principal discharge diagnoses) and resulted in a relatively short length of hospital stay (median, 2 days); nevertheless, primary GERD inpatient admissions were estimated to cost more than $380 million annually. GERD-related inpatient costs account for approximately 30% of all direct costs associated with GERD treatment.[21]

Diagnostic procedure costs

Diagnosis of GERD can usually be made based on patient history or an empiric trial of acid suppression; however, diagnostic procedures are available if a clear diagnosis continues to be in question. **Table 1** lists relevant procedure reimbursement ranges based on Medicare data in 2012. Nearly 7 million esophagogastroduodenoscopies (EGDs) are performed annually in the United States in adults,[23] and 20% to 30% are performed for the indication of reflux symptoms or GERD.[22,24] Using data from the Clinical Outcomes Research Initiative's National Endoscopic Database from

Table 1
2012 Medicare reimbursement range (minimum and maximum) for GERD-related diagnostic procedures

Procedure	Minimum Price (Facility)	Maximum Price (Nonfacility)
Diagnostic EGD	$353	$917
EGD with biopsy	$353	$917
Bravo pH	$74	$667
Ambulatory esophageal intraluminal impedance monitoring	$45	$261
Esophageal manometry	$59	$240

Abbreviation: EGD, esophagogastroduodenoscopy.
Data from Francis DO, Rymer JA, Slaughter JC, et al. High economic burden of caring for patients with suspected extraesophageal reflux. Am J Gastroenterol 2013;108:905–11.

2005 to 2010, Peery and colleagues[22] reported that 23.9% of EGDs listed reflux symptoms as an indication, and 1.2% and 5.1% listed Barrett's esophagus screening and surveillance, respectively, as indications for the procedure. Prevalence and cost information of upper endoscopies in 2009 was estimated using the Thompson Reuters MarketScan commercial (Thompson Reuters, New York, NY), Medicare, and Medicaid databases, and the total outpatient cost in the United States was found to be around $12.3 billion for upper endoscopies.[22] Assuming only 20% of these are done for indication of GERD, the direct annual cost to society of EGDs in patients with GERD can be estimated at more than $2 billion.[23]

Pharmaceutical costs

Studies have shown that pharmaceutical costs were responsible for most of the direct health care costs from GERD.[20,21] In 2004, PPI sales in the United States were in excess of $10 billion and two of the top five selling drugs in the United States were PPIs.[25] Of the 10 costliest prescription drugs from retail pharmacies for digestive diseases according to the 2004 Verispan database of retail pharmacy sales, the top five were PPIs. They constituted 50.7% of total number of prescriptions for digestive diseases and 77.3% of total costs.[21] Pharmacotherapy for GERD includes brand-name, generic, and over-the-counter antireflux medications that rank near the top of their respective lists in terms of expenditure (**Fig. 4**).[26] Any effort to substantially reduce the financial burden of GERD must be aimed at reducing the costs of medical therapy.

Despite efforts to reduce unnecessary PPI therapy, PPI overuse has been documented in several studies for inpatient and outpatient settings.[26–30] A recent study reported that a large portion of patients (42%) continue using a PPI after negative results from physiologic testing for reflux disease.[31]

Extraesophageal reflux

Many symptoms outside of the gastrointestinal tract including ear, nose, throat, pulmonary, and allergic conditions have been increasingly attributed to gastroesophageal reflux. Francis and colleagues[32] estimated the economic burden associated with such symptoms of extraesophageal reflux at a single center between 2007 and 2011. The most common diagnostic procedures performed included EGD, pulmonary function testing, wireless pH testing, and sinus computed tomography. The mean initial year direct cost was found to be more than $5000 dollars per patient being evaluated for extraesophageal reflux, significantly higher than the annual cost of typical GERD. Pharmaceuticals accounted for 86% (61% attributable to PPI use) of the total direct cost.[32]

Indirect Costs of GERD

Based on a proprietary database that contained workplace absence, disability, and workers' compensation data in addition to prescription drug and medical claims, Joish and colleagues[33] estimated a mean work absence attributed to sick days of 2.8 ($\pm$2.3) for control subjects, 3.4 ($\pm$2.5) for GERD, and 3.2 ($\pm$2.6) for peptic ulcer disease. The authors estimated that the incremental economic impact projected to a hypothetical employed population of $3441 for GERD per employee per year compared with employees without disease.

A decrease in work productivity of 41%, including time lost from work for physician visits or because of illness and reduced productivity while at work due to illness, was reported by a sample of 150 patients with GERD randomly selected from a large US health maintenance organization during a 6-month period.[34] The estimated value of lost work productivity for GERD was $237 per working subject over a 3-month period,

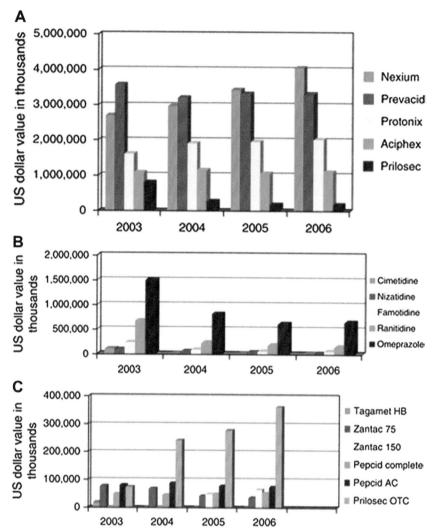

Fig. 4. (A) Total expenditure in US dollars for brand-name proton pump inhibitors in the United States from 2003 to 2006 (in thousands). (B) Total expenditure in US dollars for generic proton pump inhibitors in the United States from 2003 to 2006 (in thousands). (C) Total expenditure in US dollars for over-the-counter proton pump inhibitors in the United States from 2003 to 2006 (in thousands). (From Heidelbaugh JJ, Goldberg KL, Inadomi JM. Overutilization of proton pump inhibitors: a review of cost-effectiveness and risk in PPI. Am J Gastroenterol 2009;104:S28; with permission.)

mostly caused by time off for physician visits and reduced productivity at work. Because of the high prevalence of GERD, the loss in productivity costs from GERD can be substantial.

Productivity and quality of life have been inversely correlated with severity of GERD symptoms. Wahlqvist and colleagues[35] used a self-reported productivity instrument, the Work Productivity and Activity Impairment questionnaire (WPAI), in a population of Swedish patients with symptoms of GERD. As symptom severity increased, work productivity decreased from 16% in patients with mild GERD symptoms to 32% in patients with severe symptoms. Dean and colleagues[36] conducted a survey using the WPAI-GERD questionnaire in a sample of more than 1000 employed individuals reporting chronic heartburn. More than 30% of chronic heartburn sufferers reported reduced productivity with the proportion reporting decreased productivity correlating with disease severity. A GERD-related reduction in productivity while at work was found to be around 7.5% to 10%.[37,38] Another recent study based on more than 10,000 US respondents to the Internet-based 2004 National Health and Wellness Survey with self-reported GERD showed a correlation between increasing severity and frequency of GERD and lower health-related quality of life, measured using the Short-Form 8 survey, and lower work productivity, measured using the WPAI questionnaire.[38] The authors estimated the indirect costs of GERD including a combination of productivity costs as a result of absenteeism and reduced productivity at work and found it to account for 63% of the calculated total cost of GERD. Health care costs accounted for the remaining 37%. Costs per employed GERD respondent per month were $113 for absenteeism and $283 for reduction in productivity while at work based on their later study.[38]

RISK FACTORS FOR GERD

There is no clear association of age or gender with GERD symptoms, but advancing age, male gender, and white race are associated with the risk of GERD complications. Reports of the association between GERD symptoms and gender have yielded conflicting results, with some suggesting the prevalence is greater in men,[4,39,40] some suggesting it is greater in women,[41] and others reporting no difference by gender.[42–44] Some reports have suggested GERD symptoms are associated with age,[39–41,44] but others have suggested no association.[42,43] In contrast, mortality from GERD is associated with male gender and white race.[5] In particular, esophageal adenocarcinoma is associated with advancing age, male gender, and white race.[45]

Observational studies assessing the association between behaviors and GERD symptoms need to be interpreted cautiously. If there is a strong causal effect with little time lag between the behavior and GERD symptoms, observational studies may identify spurious inverse associations because individuals are likely to avoid the culprit behavior. For instance, alcohol consumption has been inversely associated with GERD symptoms in some surveys,[44,46,47] but physiologic studies also indicate that alcohol consumption actually worsens esophageal acid exposure.[48] However, multiple studies have demonstrated a positive association between tobacco smoking and GERD symptoms,[44,46,47] but studies of smoking cessation have not demonstrated a benefit on GERD symptoms.[48] This may be caused by an enduring effect of tobacco exposure on weakening the lower esophageal sphincter.[49]

Obesity is a strong risk factor for GERD and its complications, and might explain some of the rise in prevalence of GERD symptoms and incidence of complications (see the article on GERD and the obesity epidemic elsewhere in this issue) (**Box 1**). Some of the effect of obesity on GERD might be confounded by associated differences in physical activity or dietary patterns. Bearing in mind the issues raised previously regarding interpretation of observational studies of behavior on GERD symptoms, it seems that dietary patterns might partially confound the association of obesity with GERD. For instance, obese individuals are more likely to consume large meals with high fat intake, which can promote GERD. GERD has been positively associated with consumption of fat, sweets, chocolate, and salt, and inversely associated with consumption of fruits and fiber.[44,47,50,51] Leisure exercise is also inversely

Box 1
Risk factors for GERD

- Obesity +
- Physical activity
  - Weight lifting +
  - Frequent leisure activity −
- Diet
  - Fat +
  - Chocolate +
  - Fiber −
- Alcohol +?
- Smoking +
- Disturbed sleep +
- Respiratory disease +

associated with the presence of GERD symptoms.[44,46,47] However, physical activity at work may be positively associated with GERD symptoms.[46] The discrepancy might be related to the type of physical activity performed at work or at leisure because certain forms of physical activity (eg, weight lifting) might promote immediate GERD events.[52,53]

Infection with *Helicobacter pylori* seems to be protective against esophageal adenocarcinoma.[54] Initial reports also suggested that eradication of *H pylori* was associated with the subsequent development of GERD.[55,56] It was hypothesized that *H pylori*–induced corpus atrophy led to a decrease in gastric acid production, and hence the infection prevented GERD in people who would otherwise be predisposed.[57] However, a meta-analysis of trials of *H pylori* eradication found that there was no such increased risk of GERD symptoms after eradication of *H pylori*.[58] In some observational studies, there has been an inverse association of *H pylori* with GERD symptoms or erosive esophagitis, but the effect seems to be strongest in the Far East, where *H pylori* infection is more commonly associated with corpus atrophy than in Western countries.[59] Antral-predominant gastritis is more common in Western countries, and can be associated with an increase in gastric acid production.[60,61] In a cross-sectional study of older American men, we recently confirmed an inverse association between *H pylori* and Barrett's esophagus and erosive esophagitis, but could not detect such an association with GERD symptoms.[62] There may be other mechanisms by which *H pylori* protects against erosive esophagitis, Barrett's esophagus, and esophageal adenocarcinoma independent of any effect on GERD.

GERD is associated with other medical conditions. Most individuals with GERD symptoms do not present to a physician for management of their symptoms. Those who do present are more likely to have irritable bowel syndrome, depression, anxiety, somatization, and obsessing personalities.[63,64] GERD has also been associated with respiratory diseases, including asthma, chronic obstructive pulmonary disease, interstitial lung disease, and sleep apnea.[65–67] In each of these respiratory diseases, most of the initial work focused on how GERD might promote the respiratory complication, but at least for asthma, it seems that the predominant direction of the effect is actually from asthma on GERD.[68] Further work is needed to understand which direction the effect is with chronic obstructive pulmonary disease and interstitial lung disease. Sleep apnea represents a special case. It has long been understood that GERD can interfere with sleep, and that nocturnal symptoms increase the risk for complications. It is also becoming clear that sleep disturbance of any sort can worsen GERD symptoms by increasing esophageal sensitivity to acid.[69] Therefore, in addition to its mechanical effect promoting GERD, sleep apnea might promote esophageal hypersensitivity through sleep deprivation. Although multiple observational studies have detected an association between GERD symptoms and disturbed sleep, it is unclear whether the predominant direction of the effect is from GERD on disturbed sleep or if it is vice versa.[70–72]

SUMMARY

The prevalence of GERD symptoms rose until the mid-1990s, and then plateaued, coinciding with the market release of PPIs. Complications from GERD may also be reaching a plateau. GERD is responsible for the greatest direct costs in the United States of any gastrointestinal disease, and most of those expenditures are for pharmacotherapy. Risk factors for GERD include obesity, poor diet, lack of leisure physical activity, consumption of tobacco and alcohol, and respiratory diseases.

REFERENCES

1. Vakil N, van Zanten SV, Kahrilas P, et al, Global Consensus Group. The Montreal definition and classification of gastroesophageal reflux disease: a global evidence-based consensus. Am J Gastroenterol 2006;101:1900–20 [quiz: 43].
2. El-Serag HB. Time trends of gastroesophageal reflux disease: a systematic review. Clin Gastroenterol Hepatol 2007;5:17–26.
3. El-Serag HB, Sweet S, Winchester CC, et al. Update on the epidemiology of gastro-oesophageal reflux disease: a systematic review. Gut 2013. http://dx. doi.org/10.1136/gutjnl-2012-304269.
4. Ness-Jensen E, Lindam A, Lagergren J, et al. Changes in prevalence, incidence and spontaneous loss of gastro-oesophageal reflux symptoms: a prospective population-based cohort study, the HUNT study. Gut 2012;61:1390–7.
5. El-Serag HB, Sonnenberg A. Opposing time trends of peptic ulcer and reflux disease. Gut 1998;43:327–33.
6. Guda NM, Vakil N. Proton pump inhibitors and the time trends for esophageal dilation. Am J Gastroenterol 2004;99:797–800.
7. El-Serag HB. Temporal trends in new and recurrent esophageal strictures in Department of Veterans Affairs. Am J Gastroenterol 2006;101:1727–33.
8. El-Serag HB, Lau M. Temporal trends in new and recurrent oesophageal strictures in a Medicare population. Aliment Pharmacol Ther 2007;25:1223–9.
9. Rubenstein JH, Taylor JB. Meta-analysis: the association of oesophageal adenocarcinoma with symptoms of gastro-oesophageal reflux. Aliment Pharmacol Ther 2010;32:1222–7.
10. Blot WJ, Devesa SS, Kneller RW, et al. Rising incidence of adenocarcinoma of the esophagus and gastric cardia. JAMA 1991;265:1287–9.
11. Pohl H, Sirovich B, Welch HG. Esophageal adenocarcinoma incidence: are we reaching the peak? Cancer Epidemiol Biomarkers Prev 2010;19:1468–70.
12. Bollschweiler E, Wolfgarten E, Gutschow C, et al. Demographic variations in the rising incidence of esophageal adenocarcinoma in white males. Cancer 2001; 92:549–55.

13. Edgren G, Adami HO, Weiderpass Vainio E, et al. A global assessment of the oesophageal adenocarcinoma epidemic. Gut 2013;62(10):1406–14.
14. Rubenstein JH, Scheiman JM, Sadeghi S, et al. Esophageal adenocarcinoma incidence in individuals with gastroesophageal reflux: synthesis and estimates from population studies. Am J Gastroenterol 2011;106:254–60.
15. Hur C, Miller M, Kong CY, et al. Trends in esophageal adenocarcinoma incidence and mortality. Cancer 2013;119:1149–58.
16. van Soest EM, Dieleman JP, Siersema PD, et al. Increasing incidence of Barrett's oesophagus in the general population. Gut 2005;54:1062–6.
17. Corley DA, Kubo A, Levin TR, et al. Race, ethnicity, sex and temporal differences in Barrett's oesophagus diagnosis: a large community-based study, 1994-2006. Gut 2009;58:182–8.
18. Zagari RM, Fuccio L, Wallander MA, et al. Gastro-oesophageal reflux symptoms, oesophagitis and Barrett's oesophagus in the general population: the Loiano-Monghidoro study. Gut 2008;57:1354–9.
19. Ronkainen J, Aro P, Storskrubb T, et al. Prevalence of Barrett's esophagus in the general population: an endoscopic study. Gastroenterology 2005;129:1825–31.
20. Sandler RS, Everhart JE, Donowitz M, et al. The burden of selected digestive diseases in the United States. Gastroenterology 2002;122:1500–11.
21. Everhart JE, Ruhl CE. Burden of digestive diseases in the United States. Part I: overall and upper gastrointestinal diseases. Gastroenterology 2009;136: 376–86.
22. Peery AF, Dellon ES, Lund J, et al. Burden of gastrointestinal disease in the United States: 2012 update. Gastroenterology 2012;143:1179–87.e1–3.
23. Dellon ES, Carroll CF, Allen JK, et al. A decade of increased gastrointestinal endoscopy utilization and costs in the United States, 2000-2009 (abstract). Digestive Diseases Week 2012. ASGE 67.
24. Sonnenberg A, Amorosi SL, Lacey MJ, et al. Patterns of endoscopy in the United States: analysis of data from the Centers for Medicare and Medicaid Services and the National Endoscopic Database. Gastrointest Endosc 2008;67: 489–96.
25. Shaheen NJ, Hansen RA, Morgan DR, et al. The burden of gastrointestinal and liver diseases, 2006. Am J Gastroenterol 2006;101:2128–38.
26. Heidelbaugh JJ, Goldberg KL, Inadomi JM. Overutilization of proton pump inhibitors: a review of cost-effectiveness and risk [corrected]. Am J Gastroenterol 2009;104(Suppl 2):S27–32.
27. Heidelbaugh JJ, Goldberg KL, Inadomi JM. Magnitude and economic effect of overuse of antisecretory therapy in the ambulatory care setting. Am J Manag Care 2010;16:e228–34.
28. Heidelbaugh JJ, Kim AH, Chang R, et al. Overutilization of proton-pump inhibitors: what the clinician needs to know. Therap Adv Gastroenterol 2012;5: 219–32.
29. Heidelbaugh JJ, Metz DC, Yang YX. Proton pump inhibitors: are they overutilised in clinical practice and do they pose significant risk? Int J Clin Pract 2012;66:582–91.
30. Pasina L, Nobili A, Tettamanti M, et al. Prevalence and appropriateness of drug prescriptions for peptic ulcer and gastro-esophageal reflux disease in a cohort of hospitalized elderly. Eur J Intern Med 2011;22:205–10.
31. Gawron AJ, Rothe J, Fought AJ, et al. Many patients continue using proton pump inhibitors after negative results from tests for reflux disease. Clin Gastroenterol Hepatol 2012;10:620–5 [quiz: e57].

32. Francis DO, Rymer JA, Slaughter JC, et al. High economic burden of caring for patients with suspected extraesophageal reflux. Am J Gastroenterol 2013;108: 905–11.

33. Joish VN, Donaldson G, Stockdale W, et al. The economic impact of GERD and PUD: examination of direct and indirect costs using a large integrated employer claims database. Curr Med Res Opin 2005;21:535–44.

34. Henke CJ, Levin TR, Henning JM, et al. Work loss costs due to peptic ulcer disease and gastroesophageal reflux disease in a health maintenance organization. Am J Gastroenterol 2000;95:788–92.

35. Wahlqvist P, Carlsson J, Stalhammar NO, et al. Validity of a work productivity and activity impairment questionnaire for patients with symptoms of gastroesophageal reflux disease (WPAI-GERD): results from a cross-sectional study. Value Health 2002;5:106–13.

36. Dean BB, Crawley JA, Schmitt CM, et al. The burden of illness of gastro-oesophageal reflux disease: impact on work productivity. Aliment Pharmacol Ther 2003;17:1309–17.

37. Wahlqvist P, Reilly MC, Barkun A. Systematic review: the impact of gastro-oesophageal reflux disease on work productivity. Aliment Pharmacol Ther 2006;24:259–72.

38. Wahlqvist P, Karlsson M, Johnson D, et al. Relationship between symptom load of gastro-oesophageal reflux disease and health-related quality of life, work productivity, resource utilization and concomitant diseases: survey of a US cohort. Aliment Pharmacol Ther 2008;27:960–70.

39. Li YM, Du J, Zhang H, et al. Epidemiological investigation in outpatients with symptomatic gastroesophageal reflux from the Department of Medicine in Zhejiang Province, east China. J Gastroenterol Hepatol 2008;23:283–9.

40. Wong BC, Kinoshita Y. Systematic review on epidemiology of gastroesophageal reflux disease in Asia. Clin Gastroenterol Hepatol 2006;4:398–407.

41. Yamagishi H, Koike T, Ohara S, et al. Prevalence of gastroesophageal reflux symptoms in a large unselected general population in Japan. World J Gastroenterol 2008;14:1358–64.

42. Locke GR III, Talley NJ, Fett SL, et al. Prevalence and clinical spectrum of gastroesophageal reflux: a population-based study in Olmsted County, Minnesota. Gastroenterology 1997;112:1448–56.

43. Nouraie M, Razjouyan H, Assady M, et al. Epidemiology of gastroesophageal reflux symptoms in Tehran, Iran: a population-based telephone survey. Arch Iran Med 2007;10:289–94.

44. Nocon M, Labenz J, Willich SN. Lifestyle factors and symptoms of gastro-oesophageal reflux: a population-based study. Aliment Pharmacol Ther 2006; 23:169–74.

45. Trivers KF, Sabatino SA, Stewart SL, et al. Trends in esophageal cancer incidence by histology, United States, 1998-2003. Int J Cancer 2008;123: 1422–8.

46. Zheng Z, Nordenstedt H, Pedersen NL, et al. Lifestyle factors and risk for symptomatic gastroesophageal reflux in monozygotic twins. Gastroenterology 2007; 132:87–95.

47. Nilsson M, Johnsen R, Ye W, et al. Lifestyle related risk factors in the aetiology of gastro-oesophageal reflux. Gut 2004;53:1730–5.

48. Kaltenbach T, Crockett S, Gerson LB. Are lifestyle measures effective in patients with gastroesophageal reflux disease? An evidence-based approach. Arch Intern Med 2006;166:965–71.

49. Kahrilas PJ, Gupta RR. Mechanisms of acid reflux associated with cigarette smoking. Gut 1990;31:4–10.
50. El-Serag HB, Satia JA, Rabeneck L. Dietary intake and the risk of gastro-oesophageal reflux disease: a cross sectional study in volunteers. Gut 2005; 54:11–7.
51. Murphy DW, Castell DO. Chocolate and heartburn: evidence of increased esophageal acid exposure after chocolate ingestion. Am J Gastroenterol 1988;83:633–6.
52. Collings KL, Pierce Pratt F, Rodriguez-Stanley S, et al. Esophageal reflux in conditioned runners, cyclists, and weightlifters. Med Sci Sports Exerc 2003; 35:730–5.
53. Clark CS, Kraus BB, Sinclair J, et al. Gastroesophageal reflux induced by exercise in healthy volunteers. JAMA 1989;261:3599–601.
54. Rokkas T, Pistiolas D, Sechopoulos P, et al. Relationship between *Helicobacter pylori* infection and esophageal neoplasia: a meta-analysis. Clin Gastroenterol Hepatol 2007;5:1413–7.
55. Schutze K, Hentschel E, Dragosics B, et al. *Helicobacter pylori* reinfection with identical organisms: transmission by the patients' spouses. Gut 1995;36:831–3.
56. Labenz J, Blum AL, Bayerdorffer E, et al. Curing *Helicobacter pylori* infection in patients with duodenal ulcer may provoke reflux esophagitis. Gastroenterology 1997;112:1442–7.
57. Pandolfino JE, Howden CW, Kahrilas PJ. *H. pylori* and GERD: is less more? Am J Gastroenterol 2004;99:1222–5.
58. Yaghoobi M, Farrokhyar F, Yuan Y, et al. Is there an increased risk of GERD after *Helicobacter pylori* eradication? A meta-analysis. Am J Gastroenterol 2010;105: 1007–13.
59. Raghunath A, Hungin AP, Wooff D, et al. Prevalence of *Helicobacter pylori* in patients with gastro-oesophageal reflux disease: systematic review. BMJ 2003; 326:737.
60. Naylor GM, Gotoda T, Dixon M, et al. Why does Japan have a high incidence of gastric cancer? Comparison of gastritis between UK and Japanese patients. Gut 2006;55:1545–52.
61. el-Omar E, Penman I, Ardill J, et al. *Helicobacter pylori* infection and abnormalities of acid secretion in patients with duodenal ulcer disease. Gastroenterology 1995;109:681–91.
62. Rubenstein JH, Inadomi JM, Scheiman J, et al. Association between *Helicobacter pylori* and Barrett's esophagus, erosive esophagitis, and gastroesophageal reflux symptoms. Clin Gastroenterol Hepatol 2013. http://dx.doi.org/10. 1016/j.cgh.2013.08.029.
63. Ruigomez A, Wallander MA, Johansson S, et al. Irritable bowel syndrome and gastroesophageal reflux disease in primary care: is there a link? Dig Dis Sci 2009;54:1079–86.
64. Hungin AP, Hill C, Raghunath A. Systematic review: frequency and reasons for consultation for gastro-oesophageal reflux disease and dyspepsia. Aliment Pharmacol Ther 2009;30:331–42.
65. Havemann BD, Henderson CA, El-Serag HB. The association between gastro-oesophageal reflux disease and asthma: a systematic review. Gut 2007;56: 1654–64.
66. Martinez CH, Han MK. Contribution of the environment and comorbidities to chronic obstructive pulmonary disease phenotypes. Med Clin North Am 2012; 96:713–27.

67. Karkos PD, Leong SC, Benton J, et al. Reflux and sleeping disorders: a systematic review. J Laryngol Otol 2009;123:372–4.

68. Chan WW, Chiou E, Obstein KL, et al. The efficacy of proton pump inhibitors for the treatment of asthma in adults: a meta-analysis. Arch Intern Med 2011;171: 620–9.

69. Schey R, Dickman R, Parthasarathy S, et al. Sleep deprivation is hyperalgesic in patients with gastroesophageal reflux disease. Gastroenterology 2007;133: 1787–95.

70. Fass R, Quan SF, O'Connor GT, et al. Predictors of heartburn during sleep in a large prospective cohort study. Chest 2005;127:1658–66.

71. Zhang J, Lam SP, Li SX, et al. The longitudinal course and impact of non-restorative sleep: a five-year community-based follow-up study. Sleep Med 2012;13:570–6.

72. Matsuki N, Fujita T, Watanabe N, et al. Lifestyle factors associated with gastroesophageal reflux disease in the Japanese population. J Gastroenterol 2013;48: 340–9.

Pathophysiology of Gastroesophageal Reflux Disease

Guy E. Boeckxstaens, MD, PhD[a],*, Wout O. Rohof, MD, PhD[b]

KEYWORDS

- Gastroesophageal reflux disease • Pathophysiology • Esophagogastric junction
- Esophageal sphincter

KEY POINTS

- The high-pressure zone at the esophagogastric junction is generated by the lower esophageal sphincter (LES) and the crural diaphragm.
- Transient LES relaxations are prolonged relaxations of the LES and are the main mechanism underlying gastroesophageal reflux.
- The acid pocket is the source of postprandial acid refluxate; the position of the acid pocket relative to the diaphragm is a major determinant of the acidity of the refluxate.
- Especially in patients with nonerosive reflux disease, increased permeability and dilated intercellular spaces may contribute to symptom generation.

INTRODUCTION

Although reflux of gastric contents into the esophagus is a physiologic phenomenon, increased exposure or increased perception of the refluxate may cause troublesome symptoms and/or complications, referred to as *gastroesophageal reflux disease* (GERD).[1] GERD is one of the most common digestive diseases in the Western world, with typical symptoms, such as heartburn, regurgitation, or retrosternal pain, reported by 15% to 20% of the general population.[2] Most patients have mild to moderate complaints, but increased exposure of the esophageal epithelium to noxious gastric contents may lead to complications, such as erosive esophagitis, Barrett esophagus, peptic strictures, and even esophageal carcinoma.[3,4] The different phenotypes of GERD range from nonerosive reflux disease (NERD), through reflux esophagitis and Barrett esophagus; but most patients have no abnormalities on endoscopic

[a] Department of Gastroenterology, Translational Research Center for Gastrointestinal Disorders (TARGID), University Hospital of Leuven, University of Leuven, Herestraat 49, Leuven 3000, Belgium; [b] Department of Gastroenterology and Hepatology, Academic Medical Center, Meibergdreef 9, 1105 AZ Amsterdam, The Netherlands
* Corresponding author.
E-mail address: guy.boeckxstaens@med.kuleuven.be

Gastroenterol Clin N Am 43 (2014) 15–25
http://dx.doi.org/10.1016/j.gtc.2013.11.001
0889-8553/14/$ – see front matter © 2014 Elsevier Inc. All rights reserved.

examination. Clearly, symptoms related to GERD have to be related to reflux events.[5] This relationship depends on the presence of pathologic acid exposure during 24-hour pH-metry and a positive association between symptoms and esophageal reflux episodes. In the absence of these features, patients are rather considered to suffer from functional heartburn, a functional disorder that does not belong to the GERD spectrum.

Given the high prevalence of GERD, understanding of the pathophysiology is of great importance in order to efficiently treat our patients. In this article, the authors review the major mechanisms involved in gastroesophageal reflux.

THE ESOPHAGOGASTRIC JUNCTION

The junction between the esophagus and stomach is a highly specialized region, composed of the lower esophageal sphincter (LES) and crural diaphragm.[6] Together these structures have to reassure that a bolus of food can enter into the stomach. Conversely, reflux of gastric contents across the esophagogastric junction (EGJ) into the esophagus should be prevented, with the exception of a retrograde flow of gastric contents during vomiting or venting of accumulated air during belching.[7]

The LES is a specialized thickened region of the circular muscle layer of the distal esophagus, extending over an axial distance of 3 to 4 cm. By generating a myogenic tonic resting pressure higher than the intragastric pressure, the LES provides sufficient protection against the pressure gradient between the stomach and the intrathoracic esophagus.[7] However, during straining and inspiration, this gradient increases, requiring an additional compensatory mechanism. This task is fulfilled by the crural diaphragm, which is considered the second sphincteric component of the EGJ.[6,8] The crural diaphragm forms a canal through which the esophagus enters the abdomen and is anchored to the LES by the phrenoesophageal ligament. Since the two components are anatomically superimposed, contraction of the striated muscle of the crural diaphragm during inspiration or straining exerts pressure on the LES, leading to a dynamic and powerful increase in EGJ pressure.[6] Hence, the LES and crural diaphragm are considered the internal and external sphincter of the EGJ acting in concert to prevent gastroesophageal reflux.[8,9] Under normal conditions, the EGJ fulfills this task very efficiently, except during transient LES relaxations (TLESRs) and when both sphincters (LES and crural diaphragm) are anatomically separated as in patients with a hiatal hernia.

TLESRs

TLESRs are the predominant mechanisms underlying gastroesophageal reflux, both in normal subjects and in patients with GERD.[10,11] A TLESR is a vago-vagally mediated motor pattern triggered by the activation of vagal afferents in the cardia of the stomach by various stimuli, of which gastric distension is the most important.[12] In response to gastric distention, vagal afferents are activated triggering neurons in the dorsal motor nucleus of the vagus nerve to initiate the specific motor pattern underlying TLESRs (Fig. 1). TLESRs are characterized by a rapid relaxation of the LES, esophageal shortening, and the inhibition of the crural diaphragm, thought to be the physiologic mechanism by which the stomach vents gas.[13] The frequency of TLESRs in patients with GERD is not different from that of normal subjects.[14] However, the occurrence of acid reflux during a TLESR is twice as high in patients with GERD, especially in those with a hiatal hernia compared with healthy controls.[15] The potential explanation for this observation is discussed later.

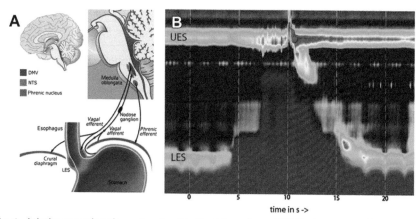

time in s ->

Fig. 1. (*A*) The neural pathway involved in the triggering of TLESRs is presented. In response to gastric distention, vagal afferents in the stomach wall are activated triggering neurons in the dorsal motor nucleus of the vagus nerve to initiate the specific motor pattern underlying TLESRs. TLESRs are characterized by a rapid relaxation of the LES, esophageal shortening, and inhibition of the crural diaphragm. (*B*) A TLESR accompanied by a liquid reflux episode is demonstrated in a high-resolution impedance manometry topography. The LES relaxes, and the rhythmic crural diaphragm contractions are inhibited. Then, a reflux episode illustrated by the purple impedance contour occurs reaching the proximal esophagus. A swallow followed by a peristaltic contraction terminates the TLESR. DMV, dorsal motor nucleus of the vagal nerve; NTS, nucleus of the solitary tract; UES, upper esophageal sphincter.

Hiatal Hernia

In healthy people, the distal part of the lower esophageal sphincter is located in the abdomen and the crural diaphragm is superimposed, leading to a synergistic high pressure zone. In the presence of a hiatal hernia, the capacity of the EGJ to prevent reflux is hampered, mainly because the stomach has migrated more proximal through the diaphragmatic hiatus into the mediastinum separating the high-pressure zones of the LES and the crural diaphragm. In addition, the hiatal sac may function as a reservoir from which fluid can re-reflux into the esophagus after swallowing or during periods of low sphincter pressure.[16]

A hiatal hernia is associated with more severe erosive esophagitis and Barrett esophagus.[17–19] This increase in esophageal injury is caused by a prolonged acid exposure time, which in its turn results from a larger number of reflux episodes in patients with hiatal hernia than in those without, and a prolonged acid clearance time.[18,19] In contrast to earlier thoughts, a hiatal hernia is a dynamic entity. A recent study clearly showed that a hiatal hernia can be intermittent as a result of axial movement of the LES through the diaphragmatic hiatus. Most intriguingly, the rate of reflux episodes is almost doubled when the hiatal hernia is present compared with periods when the hiatal hernia is absent, further illustrating the importance of hiatal hernia in GERD.[20] The increase in reflux episodes in patients with a hiatal hernia is mainly explained by the observation that, in addition to TLESRs, other mechanisms come into play. Indeed, half of the reflux episodes in patients with GERD with a hiatal hernia occur during swallowing or straining.[21] Moreover, during spatial separation, the rate of acid reflux episodes during a TLESR is doubled compared with the rate without spatial separation,[20] most likely because of the alteration of the position of the gastric acid pocket.

Acid Pocket

Most reflux episodes occur after a meal, when the stomach is filled with food, known to trigger TLESRs. In contrast to the thought that meal ingestion buffers gastric acid, acid reflux episodes occur even in the early postprandial period.[22] Fletcher and colleagues[23] elegantly showed that gastric acid floats on top of the meal acting as a reservoir from which acid can enter the esophagus during episodes of opening of the EGJ. Using a gradual pull-through pH-metry, they discovered a highly acidic zone of approximately 2 cm near the EGJ in the postprandial state. This gastric acid pocket accounted for the lower pH of the refluxate compared with the gastric postprandial pH.[23]

Recently, the existence of the acid pocket was confirmed using scintigraphy in both healthy subjects and patients with GERD.[24] Patients with GERD have larger acid pockets, whereas the proximal extent of the acid pocket is closer to the LES in patients than in healthy subjects. Most importantly, Beaumont and colleagues[22] demonstrated that the major risk factor for acid reflux is the presence of a hiatal hernia and the position of the acid pocket relative to the diaphragm (**Fig. 2**). Clearly, if the acid pocket extends into the hiatal opening or is located above the diaphragm, the pocket is the major source of refluxate, resulting in a 5-fold increased risk of having acid reflux.[22] Moreover, in patients with a large hiatal hernia it was demonstrated that the hiatal sac can function as a reservoir from which fluid can re-reflux into the esophagus during swallowing and straining.[16,22,25] This finding explains the increased risk to have acidic gastroesophageal reflux during a TLESR, when the LES relaxes after swallowing or when LES pressure is low in patients with a hiatal hernia.[24]

Prokinetic agents, such as azithromycin, increase proximal tone and promote gastric emptying. Because of this prokinetic effect, azithromycin displaces the acid pocket to a more distal location in patients with GERD with a small hiatal hernia. This more distally located acid pocket leads to less frequent postprandial acid reflux

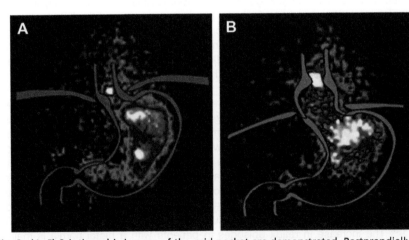

Fig. 2. (*A, B*) Scintigraphic images of the acid pocket are demonstrated. Postprandially, the acid pocket is formed and located in the proximal stomach floating on top of the ingested food. In healthy volunteers and most patients without a hiatal hernia, the acid pocket is located below the crural diaphragm (*A*). If the acid pocket is located below the diaphragm, the risk for acid reflux is low (10%–20%). In contrast, if the acid pocket is located in the hiatal sac and, thus, above the crural diaphragm (*B*), the risk for acidic reflux is very high (90%–95%).

episodes compared with placebo.[26] An alternative approach to prokinetics is the use of alginates. Alginates are natural polysaccharide polymers that, after contact with gastric acid, precipitate into a low-density viscous gel or raft of near-neutral pH in a matter of seconds. This alginate-antacid raft formed after ingestion colocalizes with the postprandial acid pocket and displaces it below the diaphragm, resulting in significant suppression of postprandial acid reflux.[27] Hence, the acid pocket is considered an interesting target for treatment, mainly because it represents the reservoir from which reflux seems to occur.[28]

Positive Pressure Gradient and Obesity

Retrograde flow across the EGJ requires a positive pressure gradient between the stomach and the distal esophagus.[29] It is well accepted that abdominal straining, for example, induces reflux if the generated pressures is higher that the EGJ pressure. In line with this, ambulatory manometric recordings in patients with GERD indeed reveal that straining occurs at the onset of 31% of acid reflux episodes.[30] Obesity, on the other hand, leads to a chronically increased pressure gradient and has been abundantly demonstrated as a risk factor for GERD.[31] In fact, the rising prevalence of GERD has, in part, been attributed to the rapidly increasing prevalence of obesity.[32] In a recent study, Lee and colleagues[33] demonstrated that central obesity causes partial hiatus herniation and short-segment acid reflux, providing a plausible explanation for the high incidence of inflammation and metaplasia and occurrence of neoplasia at the EGJ.[34,35] This finding explains how obesity increases the risk of reflux symptoms, prolonged esophageal acid exposure, esophagitis, and Barrett esophagus, further emphasizing that increased abdominal pressure is a pivotal mechanistic factor.[33,34]

Gastric Motility

Delayed gastric emptying is observed more often in patients with GERD compared with healthy volunteers as demonstrated in a recent systematic review by Penagini and Bravi.[30] However, a relationship between delayed gastric emptying and increased esophageal acid exposure has not been convincingly demonstrated.[30] Moreover, dyspepsia, regurgitation, or dysphagia, symptoms associated with delayed gastric emptying, have no differentiating value in patients with GERD.[36] Taken together, these data suggest that impaired gastric emptying is not a major factor in the pathophysiology of GERD.

Esophageal Clearance

When refluxate reaches the esophagus, clearance is mainly mediated by esophageal peristalsis, triggered by mechanoreceptors in the esophageal lumen, and gravity accounting for approximately 95%.[37] Subsequently, salivary bicarbonate further contributes to acid clearance by neutralizing the acid and normalizing esophageal pH. Obviously, rapid clearance of acid from the esophagus is crucial because prolonged clearance is associated with the development of esophagitis and Barrett metaplasia.[32] In line, impaired refluxate clearance caused by the supine position, a lack in secondary peristalsis, and reduced saliva production during sleep[38] explains the increased severity of erosive esophagitis observed in cases of nocturnal reflux.[39] Similarly, prolonged esophageal clearance in esophageal motility disorders, such as in weak or absent peristalsis, carries an increased risk to develop esophagitis and reflux symptoms.[40]

PERCEPTION OF REFLUX EPISODES

Typical reflux symptoms (ie, heartburn and regurgitation) arise because of the reflux of gastric content into the esophagus. However, the relation between magnitude and onset of reflux and symptom generation in patients with GERD is far from simple. Using 24-hour pH and multi-intraluminal impedance monitoring, Bredenoord and colleagues[41] showed in patients with GERD off proton pump inhibitors (PPIs) that symptoms only occurred during 203 of 1807 reflux episodes (11%). The possible factors that increase the likelihood of perception are episodes with a larger pH decrease, a high proximal extent of the refluxate, a lower nadir pH, and a longer clearance time.[41] Similarly, in patients with persistent symptoms during acid suppressive therapy, only 468 of 3547 (13%) reflux episodes were symptomatic.[42] Reflux episodes reaching the proximal esophagus were more likely to cause symptoms compared with those reaching the distal esophagus only.

The actual symptom perception of the esophagus occurs in the central nervous system and differs widely between patients and in patients in time. The sensory innervation of the esophagus is supplied by vagal and spinal afferents, where the spinal afferents mainly transport the painful stimuli. Peripheral afferent nerve endings contain chemoreceptors, mechanoreceptors, and thermoreceptors, allowing the perception of stimuli from the esophageal lumen.[43] Several channels are sensitive to low pH in the esophagus. These channels include the transient receptor potential vanilloid subtype 1 (TRPV-1) and the acid-sensing ion (ASIC). Increased perception or visceral hypersensitivity can result from sensitization of peripheral nerves, sensitization of spinal cord dorsal horn neurons, or interactions via the psychoneuroimmune system.[43] Especially in patients with NERD with a normal refluxate exposure, visceral hypersensitivity is of eminent importance.

Peripheral Sensitization

In response to excessive noxious stimuli (acid, pepsin, bile) inflammatory mediators, such as ATP, bradykinin, prostaglandins, histamine, and hydrochloric acid, are released. Because of these inflammatory mediators, the threshold of transduction of the peripheral receptors on vagal and spinal afferents (nociceptors) is reduced. This reduced threshold results in increased permeability of the pain receptor cation channels and primary hyperalgesia.[43] Subsequently, several nociceptors, such as the TRPV-1, in nerve fibers and other proton-gated ion channels, such as ASICs and P2X purinergic receptors, are upregulated.[43–45] This upregulation has been demonstrated in patients with reflux esophagitis and NERD.[46,47] As reviewed by Knowles and Aziz,[43] patients with NERD have an increased response not only to acid but also to mechanical stimulation, electrical stimulation, and temperature changes. This increase in perception seems to be less pronounced in patients with reflux esophagitis or Barrett metaplasia.

Central Sensitization and Psychoneuroimmune Interactions

Repetitive painful signaling from the periphery leads to phenotypical changes in the spinal dorsal horn neurons with concurrent amplification of incoming sensory information of both noxious (hyperalgesia) and innocuous stimuli (allodynia).[43] Moreover, this so-called mechanism of central sensitization may affect adjacent spinal neurons leading to hypersensitivity in remote areas (secondary hypersensitivity), like the upper esophagus and the chest wall,[43] as observed in noncardiac chest pain.[48]

The role of stress and its influence, especially in NERD, has been widely investigated. Patients with stress are more likely to have symptoms, even in the absence of increased reflux.[49] Moreover, recurrent symptoms after acid suppression are more common in patients with psychological distress.[50] Both auditory stress and sleep deprivation have been shown to influence the perception of heartburn symptoms, making the role of the central nervous system eminent in this process.[51,52] Sleep deprivation and auditory stress lower the initial time of symptoms after acid infusion; however, reported symptoms are significantly more painful.

ESOPHAGEAL INJURY

Exposure of the esophagus to noxious gastric contents, including acid, pepsin, and bile, may lead to esophageal injury and heartburn. Hydrochloric acid in the gastric refluxate damages epithelial cells by disturbing the pH-ion balance.[53,54] On the other hand, pepsins affect the intercellular substance and cell membrane by their proteolytic activity.[55] However, most pepsins are inactive in a pH greater than 4; therefore, the synergism with acid is needed for pepsin to cause damage.[55] In contrast, recent studies demonstrate that small amounts of acid (or weakly acid) can also cause dilated intercellular spaces (DIS) and, thereby, lead to an impaired mucosal barrier.[56,57]

In addition to acid, bile acids have also been shown to disrupt the integrity of the esophageal mucosa. First, in view of their lipophilic state, bile acids gain entrance across the mucosa and intracellular where they cause intramucosal damage by disorganizing membrane structure or by interfering with cellular function.[58] Bile and acid have shown synergistic potential in causing esophageal injury primarily in animal models.[58] Exposure of the esophageal mucosa to bile as a result of duodenogastroesophageal reflux is associated with the highest grade of mucosal injury.[59] In contrast to these earlier studies, however, Farre and colleagues[56] observed similar changes in intercellular spaces following acid or acid and bile acid perfusion in the distal esophagus.[60] Clearly, further studies are required to elucidate the exact role of bile acids in NERD.

Esophageal Defense and Mucosal Changes

In the healthy esophagus, nociceptors are separated from noxious substances in the esophageal lumen by a tight barrier of squamous epithelium. In this epithelium, the apical membranes and junctional complexes of the cell prevent the diffusion of noxious refluxed luminal contents from penetrating into the esophageal mucosa.[61] The first and critical step in esophageal defense is esophageal clearance by peristalsis and gravity. As previously indicated, these mechanisms account for at least 95% of the refluxate clearance. If peristalsis fails to clear the refluxate, the risk of developing mucosal damage will largely depend on the endogenous defense mechanisms of the mucosa. These mechanisms consist of the following: (1) pre-epithelial, (2) the epithelium itself, and (3) postepithelial. In short, the pre-epithelial barrier consists of secreted buffers in saliva and mucus. However, the protection by this mucous layer against acid is rather limited because the refluxed acid usually has a very high load of hydrochloric acid compared with the mucosal buffering capacity.

The next line of defense is represented by the stratified squamous epithelium. The apical cell membrane in conjunction with tight junctions effectively block hydrochloric acid and other noxious agents to enter the interstitium. The typical histopathologic finding observed when the epithelium is damaged is DIS, mainly observed at transmission electron microscopy.[62] The exact mechanism by which the contents of refluxate destruct tight junctions is unknown, but a recent study suggests that the proteolytic cleavage of the tight junction protein e-cadherin accounts for the increase in mucosal permeability.[63] Other studies, however, have demonstrated that DIS are also observed when the esophagus is exposed to acid alone, even to weakly acid.[56,62] The formation of DIS may subsequently lead to an impaired mucosal barrier, as has been demonstrated in vitro and in vivo.[64] Moreover, Woodland and colleagues[57] recently demonstrated that impaired mucosal integrity in patients with GERD is associated with sensitivity to acid perfusion and GERD symptoms.[65] Taken together, these data implicate that, especially in patients with NERD, dilated esophageal spaces and impaired mucosal integrity are important factors in pathophysiology and still might be the key factors explaining why these patients have reflux symptoms.

The postepithelial defense starts at the basal membrane with an important contribution of the rich capillary blood flow. Blood contains neutralizing buffers, oxygen, inflammatory and phagocytic cells, and a route for disposal of noxious products.[66]

When the refluxate overcomes all mucosal defense mechanisms, it will lead to microscopic and macroscopic mucosal changes. Macroscopic damage comprises erosive esophagitis, Barrett esophagus, and strictures. Microscopic damage comprises basal cell hyperplasia, elongation of the papillae, increased numbers of inflammatory cells, and DIS.[67]

SUMMARY

GERD is a complex multifactorial disease. The different factors contributing to GERD include reduced LES pressure, TLESRs, hiatal hernia, acid pocket, impaired esophageal clearance, increased abdominal pressure, visceral hypersensitivity, impaired mucosal integrity, central sensitization, and psychological factors. Although our understanding of the mechanisms underlying GERD has significantly improved over recent years, it still remains unclear why patients consciously perceive more reflux episodes or, along the same line, which mechanisms trigger PPI-resistant symptoms. The discovery of the acid pocket, on the other hand, adds significantly to our understanding; but clearly more studies are needed to demonstrate its potential as a therapeutic target.

REFERENCES

1. Kahrilas PJ, Shaheen NJ, Vaezi MF, et al. American Gastroenterological Association medical position statement on the management of gastroesophageal reflux disease. Gastroenterology 2008;135:1383–91, 1391.
2. El-Serag HB, Sweet S, Winchester CC, et al. Update on the epidemiology of gastro-oesophageal reflux disease: a systematic review. Gut 2013. [Epub ahead of print].
3. Lagergren J, Bergstrom R, Lindgren A, et al. Symptomatic gastroesophageal reflux as a risk factor for esophageal adenocarcinoma. N Engl J Med 1999;340: 825–31.
4. Champion G, Richter JE, Vaezi MF, et al. Duodenogastroesophageal reflux: relationship to pH and importance in Barrett's esophagus. Gastroenterology 1994; 107:747–54.
5. Modlin IM, Hunt RH, Malfertheiner P, et al. Non-erosive reflux disease–defining the entity and delineating the management. Digestion 2008;78(Suppl 1):1–5.
6. Mittal RK, Balaban DH. The esophagogastric junction. N Engl J Med 1997;336: 924–32.
7. Boeckxstaens GE. The lower oesophageal sphincter. Neurogastroenterol Motil 2005;17(Suppl 1):13–21.
8. Mittal RK. The crural diaphragm, an external lower esophageal sphincter: a definitive study. Gastroenterology 1993;105:1565–7.

9. Miller L, Dai Q, Korimilli A, et al. Use of endoluminal ultrasound to evaluate gastrointestinal motility. Dig Dis 2006;24:319–41.
10. Dent J, Dodds WJ, Friedman RH, et al. Mechanism of gastroesophageal reflux in recumbent asymptomatic human subjects. J Clin Invest 1980;65:256–67.
11. Dodds WJ, Dent J, Hogan WJ, et al. Mechanisms of gastroesophageal reflux in patients with reflux esophagitis. N Engl J Med 1982;307:1547–52.
12. Page AJ, Blackshaw LA. An in vitro study of the properties of vagal afferent fibres innervating the ferret oesophagus and stomach. J Physiol 1998;512(Pt 3):907–16.
13. Mittal RK, Holloway RH, Penagini R, et al. Transient lower esophageal sphincter relaxation. Gastroenterology 1995;109:601–10.
14. Sifrim D, Holloway R. Transient lower esophageal sphincter relaxations: how many or how harmful? Am J Gastroenterol 2001;96:2529–32.
15. Trudgill NJ, Riley SA. Transient lower esophageal sphincter relaxations are no more frequent in patients with gastroesophageal reflux disease than in asymptomatic volunteers. Am J Gastroenterol 2001;96:2569–74.
16. Sloan S, Kahrilas PJ. Impairment of esophageal emptying with hiatal hernia. Gastroenterology 1991;100:596–605.
17. Bredenoord AJ, Hemmink GJ, Smout AJ. Relationship between gastro-oesophageal reflux pattern and severity of mucosal damage. Neurogastroenterol Motil 2009;21:807–12.
18. Jones MP, Sloan SS, Rabine JC, et al. Hiatal hernia size is the dominant determinant of esophagitis presence and severity in gastroesophageal reflux disease. Am J Gastroenterol 2001;96:1711–7.
19. Jones MP, Sloan SS, Jovanovic B, et al. Impaired egress rather than increased access: an important independent predictor of erosive oesophagitis. Neurogastroenterol Motil 2002;14:625–31.
20. Bredenoord AJ, Weusten BL, Timmer R, et al. Intermittent spatial separation of diaphragm and lower esophageal sphincter favors acidic and weakly acidic reflux. Gastroenterology 2006;130:334–40.
21. van Herwaarden MA, Samsom M, Smout AJ. Excess gastroesophageal reflux in patients with hiatus hernia is caused by mechanisms other than transient LES relaxations. Gastroenterology 2000;119:1439–46.
22. Beaumont H, Bennink RJ, de JJ, et al. The position of the acid pocket as a major risk factor for acidic reflux in healthy subjects and patients with GORD. Gut 2010;59:441–51.
23. Fletcher J, Wirz A, Young J, et al. Unbuffered highly acidic gastric juice exists at the gastroesophageal junction after a meal. Gastroenterology 2001;121:775–83.
24. Beaumont H, Boeckxstaens GE. Scintigraphic imaging of the acid pocket: an enlarged pocket with acid coating the distal esophagus in GERD patients with hiatal hernia. 2009.
25. Mittal RK, Lange RC, McCallum RW. Identification and mechanism of delayed esophageal acid clearance in subjects with hiatus hernia. Gastroenterology 1987;92:130–5.
26. Rohof WO, Bennink RJ, de Ruigh AA, et al. Effect of azithromycin on acid reflux, hiatus hernia and proximal acid pocket in the postprandial period. Gut 2012;61:1670–7.
27. Rohof WO, Bennink RJ, Smout AJ, et al. An alginate-antacid formulation localizes to the acid pocket to reduce acid reflux in patients with gastroesophageal reflux disease. Clin Gastroenterol Hepatol 2013;11(12):1585–91.
28. Kahrilas PJ, McColl K, Fox M, et al. The acid pocket: a target for treatment in reflux disease? Am J Gastroenterol 2013;108:1058–64.

29. Pandolfino JE, Zhang QG, Ghosh SK, et al. Transient lower esophageal sphincter relaxations and reflux: mechanistic analysis using concurrent fluoroscopy and high-resolution manometry. Gastroenterology 2006;131:1725–33.
30. Penagini R, Bravi I. The role of delayed gastric emptying and impaired oesophageal body motility. Best Pract Res Clin Gastroenterol 2010;24:831–45.
31. Anand G, Katz PO. Gastroesophageal reflux disease and obesity. Gastroenterol Clin North Am 2010;39:39–46.
32. Bredenoord AJ, Pandolfino JE, Smout AJ. Gastro-oesophageal reflux disease. Lancet 2013;381:1933–42.
33. Lee YY, Wirz AA, Whiting JG, et al. Waist belt and central obesity cause partial hiatus hernia and short-segment acid reflux in asymptomatic volunteers. Gut 2013. [Epub ahead of print].
34. Robertson EV, Derakhshan MH, Wirz AA, et al. Central obesity in asymptomatic volunteers is associated with increased intrasphincteric acid reflux and lengthening of the cardiac mucosa. Gastroenterology 2013;145:730–9.
35. El-Serag HB, Hashmi A, Garcia J, et al. Visceral abdominal obesity measured by CT scan is associated with an increased risk of Barrett's oesophagus: a case-control study. Gut 2013. [Epub ahead of print].
36. Buckles DC, Sarosiek I, McMillin C, et al. Delayed gastric emptying in gastroesophageal reflux disease: reassessment with new methods and symptomatic correlations. Am J Med Sci 2004;327:1–4.
37. Sarosiek J, McCallum RW. Mechanisms of oesophageal mucosal defence. Baillieres Best Pract Res Clin Gastroenterol 2000;14:701–17.
38. Orr WC, Heading R, Johnson LF, et al. Review article: sleep and its relationship to gastro-oesophageal reflux. Aliment Pharmacol Ther 2004;20(Suppl 9):39–46.
39. Adachi K, Fujishiro H, Katsube T, et al. Predominant nocturnal acid reflux in patients with Los Angeles grade C and D reflux esophagitis. J Gastroenterol Hepatol 2001;16:1191–6.
40. Kahrilas PJ, Dodds WJ, Hogan WJ. Effect of peristaltic dysfunction on esophageal volume clearance. Gastroenterology 1988;94:73–80.
41. Bredenoord AJ, Weusten BL, Curvers WL, et al. Determinants of perception of heartburn and regurgitation. Gut 2006;55:313–8.
42. Tutuian R, Vela MF, Hill EG, et al. Characteristics of symptomatic reflux episodes on acid suppressive therapy. Am J Gastroenterol 2008;103:1090–6.
43. Knowles CH, Aziz Q. Visceral hypersensitivity in non-erosive reflux disease. Gut 2008;57:674–83.
44. Weijenborg PW, Bredenoord AJ. How reflux causes symptoms: reflux perception in gastroesophageal reflux disease. Best Pract Res Clin Gastroenterol 2013;27:353–64.
45. Holzer P. Acid-sensitive ion channels in gastrointestinal function. Curr Opin Pharmacol 2003;3:618–25.
46. Matthews PJ, Aziz Q, Facer P, et al. Increased capsaicin receptor TRPV1 nerve fibres in the inflamed human oesophagus. Eur J Gastroenterol Hepatol 2004;16:897–902.
47. Bhat YM, Bielefeldt K. Capsaicin receptor (TRPV1) and non-erosive reflux disease. Eur J Gastroenterol Hepatol 2006;18:263–70.
48. Sarkar S, Aziz Q, Woolf CJ, et al. Contribution of central sensitisation to the development of non-cardiac chest pain. Lancet 2000;356:1154–9.
49. Wright CE, Ebrecht M, Mitchell R, et al. The effect of psychological stress on symptom severity and perception in patients with gastro-oesophageal reflux. J Psychosom Res 2005;59:415–24.

50. Velden vd A, de Wit NJ, Quartero AO, et al. Maintenance treatment for GERD: residual symptoms are associated with psychological distress. Digestion 2008;77:207–13.
51. Schey R, Dickman R, Parthasarathy S, et al. Sleep deprivation is hyperalgesic in patients with gastroesophageal reflux disease. Gastroenterology 2007;133: 1787–95.
52. Fass R, Naliboff BD, Fass SS, et al. The effect of auditory stress on perception of intraesophageal acid in patients with gastroesophageal reflux disease. Gastroenterology 2008;134:696–705.
53. Orlando RC, Bryson JC, Powell DW. Mechanisms of H+ injury in rabbit esophageal epithelium. Am J Physiol 1984;246:G718–24.
54. Snow JC, Goldstein JL, Schmidt LN, et al. Rabbit esophageal cells show regulatory volume decrease: ionic basis and effect of pH. Gastroenterology 1993; 105:102–10.
55. Roberts NB. Review article: human pepsins - their multiplicity, function and role in reflux disease. Aliment Pharmacol Ther 2006;24(Suppl 2):2–9.
56. Farre R, Fornari F, Blondeau K, et al. Acid and weakly acidic solutions impair mucosal integrity of distal exposed and proximal non-exposed human oesophagus. Gut 2010;59:164–9.
57. Woodland P, Al-Zinaty M, Yazaki E, et al. In vivo evaluation of acid-induced changes in oesophageal mucosa integrity and sensitivity in non-erosive reflux disease. Gut 2013;62(9):1256–61.
58. Vaezi MF, Singh S, Richter JE. Role of acid and duodenogastric reflux in esophageal mucosal injury: a review of animal and human studies. Gastroenterology 1995;108:1897–907.
59. Oh DS, Hagen JA, Fein M, et al. The impact of reflux composition on mucosal injury and esophageal function. J Gastrointest Surg 2006;10:787–96.
60. Calabrese C, Fabbri A, Bortolotti M, et al. Dilated intercellular spaces as a marker of oesophageal damage: comparative results in gastro-oesophageal reflux disease with or without bile reflux. Aliment Pharmacol Ther 2003;18:525–32.
61. Barlow WJ, Orlando RC. The pathogenesis of heartburn in nonerosive reflux disease: a unifying hypothesis. Gastroenterology 2005;128:771–8.
62. Malenstein H, Farre R, Sifrim D. Esophageal dilated intercellular spaces (DIS) and nonerosive reflux disease. Am J Gastroenterol 2008;103:1021–8.
63. Jovov B, Que J, Tobey NA, et al. Role of E-cadherin in the pathogenesis of gastroesophageal reflux disease. Am J Gastroenterol 2011;106:1039–47.
64. Tobey NA, Hosseini SS, Argote CM, et al. Dilated intercellular spaces and shunt permeability in nonerosive acid-damaged esophageal epithelium. Am J Gastroenterol 2004;99:13–22.
65. Kessing BF, Bredenoord AJ, Weijenborg PW, et al. Esophageal acid exposure decreases intraluminal baseline impedance levels. Am J Gastroenterol 2011; 106:2093–7.
66. Boeckxstaens GE. Review article: the pathophysiology of gastro-oesophageal reflux disease. Aliment Pharmacol Ther 2007;26:149–60.
67. Edebo A, Vieth M, Tam W, et al. Circumferential and axial distribution of esophageal mucosal damage in reflux disease. Dis Esophagus 2007;20:232–8.

Symptom Predictability in Gastroesophageal Reflux Disease and Role of Proton Pump Inhibitor Test

David S. Estores, MD

KEYWORDS

- Heartburn • Regurgitation • Gastroesophageal reflux/symptoms/diagnosis/
treatment • Proton pump inhibitor

KEY POINTS

- The symptoms of heartburn and regurgitation may be sensitive but are not adequately specific for diagnosing or excluding gastroesophageal reflux disease (GERD).
- Symptom assessment, particularly from a patient's perspective, is important and tools for measuring these are validated.
- The poorly defined but popular proton pump inhibitor (PPI) test is neither sensitive nor specific enough for diagnosing/excluding GERD.
- The use of the GERD outcomes measures (Reflux Disease Questionnaire and GERD Questionnaire) may be helpful in identifying patients in primary care for whom a PPI test may be cost-effective.
- These measures may be best used as components of a clinical pathway/algorithm for GERD diagnosis/evaluation.

Heartburn and regurgitation are the most common symptoms of gastroesophageal reflux disease (GERD) and are widely accepted as the classic symptoms. Heartburn is most commonly defined as a burning, retrosternal, painful sensation of short duration associated with a meal and regurgitation is defined as the retrograde flow of presumed gastric contents or a sensation of bitter contents in the mouth without associated nausea or retching. In clinical practice, the meaning of heartburn is not standardized and well communicated. In a group of 129 patients from Boston, Spechler and colleagues[1] reported that the term heartburn was understood by only 34.6%, 53.8%, and 13.2% of white people, black people, and East Asian people, respectively.

Disclosures: None.

Division of Gastroenterology, Hepatology and Nutrition, University of Florida, PO BOX 100214, Gainesville, FL 32610-0214, USA

E-mail address: David.Estores@medicine.ufl.edu

Gastroenterol Clin N Am 43 (2014) 27–38
http://dx.doi.org/10.1016/j.gtc.2013.11.002
0889-8553/14/$ – see front matter © 2014 Elsevier Inc. All rights reserved.

In the same study, among patients who claimed that they had heartburn, 29.7% did not describe symptoms that a reasonable clinician would define as heartburn. In contrast, 22.8% of patients who denied having heartburn experienced symptoms that physicians might consider to be heartburn. Sharma and colleagues[2] recommended that both language and cultural barriers be considered in the evaluation and treatment of patients with GERD.

SYMPTOM ASSESSMENT

The accurate assessment of symptoms in GERD is of prime importance. Symptom assessment is the means by which a primary care provider or a gastroenterologist makes the initial diagnosis, assesses the severity of disease, formulates a diagnostic work-up, starts treatment if appropriate, and later assesses the response to treatment.

ISSUES IN GERD SYMPTOM ASSESSMENT

A significant issue in dealing with GERD symptom assessment is the lack of correlation between the severity of heartburn and the degree of acid exposure or mucosal damage.[3] GERD symptoms are the main causes of morbidity and negatively affect quality of life, with little additional impact of endoscopic findings such as erosions or Barrett esophagus.[4] There are gender differences among patients with GERD symptoms. These symptom differences have been described and there is evidence to show that the symptom severity in women is significantly greater than in men (**Fig. 1**).[5] This finding may account for GERD-related complications being more common in men, possibly because of lesser sensitivity to gastroesophageal reflux. There is

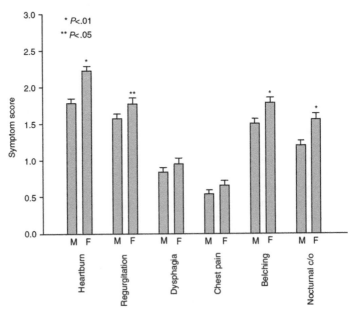

Fig. 1. Quantitative esophageal symptom analysis in women compared with men for all GERD stages (0–IV). There is a significantly higher symptom severity score for heartburn ($P<.01$), regurgitation ($P<.05$), belching ($P<.01$), and nocturnal symptoms (c/o; $P<.01$) in women (F) compared with men (M). (*From* Lin M, Gerson LB, Lascar R, et al. Features of gastroesophageal reflux disease in women. Am J Gastroenterol 2004;99(8):1442–7; with permission.)

a disparity in the assessment of GERD symptoms from the patient and physician perspectives, particularly before treatment initiation and for more severe symptoms.[6]

EVALUATION OF SYMPTOMS IN GERD

Based on data collected during a workshop in 2002 centered on symptom evaluation in reflux disease, impairment in quality of life is significant for patients who have heartburn symptoms occurring on more than 1 day of the week and whose heartburn is of moderate or greater severity.[7]

PATIENT-REPORTED OUTCOMES IN GERD SYMPTOM ASSESSMENT

In order to standardize the criteria for patient selection and evaluate response to therapy, several symptom-based GERD questionnaires (GERDQs) have been proposed, studied, and validated. There has been a shift toward patient-reported outcomes (PRO); these instruments assess disease severity from a patient's perspective.

To ensure the validity of such questionnaires, the US Food and Drug Administration (FDA) stipulated that these so-called PRO measures must have certain properties: content validity (evidence that the instrument measures what it is intended to measure), construct validity (evidence of a logical relationship between items, domains, and concepts), internal consistency (intercorrelation of items that contribute to a score), test-retest reliability (stability of scores over time when no change is expected in the concept of interest), and ability to detect change (evidence that the PRO can detect differences in scores over time when changes in the measured variable have occurred).[8] In another systematic review for PROs measures in GERD, Vakil and colleagues[9] reported that there are 5 instruments (GERD Symptom Assessment Scale, Nocturnal GERD Symptom Severity and Impact Questionnaire, Proton Pump Acid Suppression Symptom Test, Reflux Disease Questionnaire [RDQ], and Reflux Questionnaire) that include most steps recommended by the FDA and European Medicines Agency, and have been used as end point measures in clinical trials. In 2012 a systematic review by Chassany and colleagues[8] reported on the considerable heterogeneity in the methodology used to develop PRO instruments for upper gastrointestinal disease. The investigators identified 10 studies (out of an initial 94 studies before exclusion criteria were applied) reporting a symptom scale PRO instrument for GERD or dyspepsia.

Among these self-administered PRO questionnaires, the RDQ is a practical and easily administered instrument targeted for use in a primary care setting.[9] This questionnaire was used recently in the Diamond study to evaluate a cohort of patients presenting to primary care physicians in Europe and Canada.[10] This study was based on 73 family practice clinics during which an RDQ was administered to patients after recruitment into the study during the first visit. The patients were placed on daily placebo before an endoscopy and 48-hour esophageal wireless pH probe study. The patients were then started on esomeprazole 40 mg daily for 14 $\pm$ 3 days (**Fig. 2**).[10] Of the 308 evaluable patients, 203 patients (65.9%) were diagnosed with GERD from reflux esophagitis by endoscopy and/or a positive 48-hour wireless esophageal pH study. The prevalence of heartburn and regurgitation as the most common symptom in patients with GERD is 49.3% versus 25.5% in patients without GERD. The prevalence of heartburn and regurgitation as the second most common symptoms in patients with GERD is 41.8% versus 21% in patients without GERD.

The RDQ includes 12 items in which 6 symptom descriptors covering 3 symptom domains, consisting of heartburn, regurgitation, and dyspepsia (upper abdominal

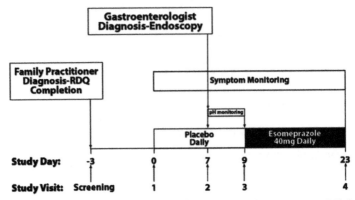

Outline of the main study interventions and their timings.

Fig. 2. Proportion of patients with relief of reflux symptoms in response to PPI day by day. (*From* Dent J, Vakil N, Jones R, et al. Accuracy of the diagnosis of GORD by questionnaire, physicians and a trial of proton pump inhibitor treatment: the Diamond Study. Gut 2010;59(6):714–21; with permission.)

pain and burning), are assessed separately for their frequency and severity in the previous 7 days, using a 6-point Liker scale As shown in **Table 1**,[10] a score of 0 is assigned to the first column, a score of 1 for the second column, and so forth. A maximum of 5 points is assigned for the most severe and frequent symptom designation. Based on receiver operating characteristic (ROC) curve for best-performing prespecified scoring method, the investigators of the Diamond study assigned negative value to responses on dyspepsia ("a burning feeling in the center of the upper stomach" and "a pain in the center of the upper stomach"). The RDQ scores range from 0 to a maximum of 30. A diagnosis of GERD based on a reflux esophagitis or a positive 48-hour wireless esophageal pH study are found in 77% of patients with an RDQ total of 15 to 19, and in 88% of patients with an RDQ total of 20 to 30 (**Fig. 3**).[10]

Another PRO questionnaire is the GERDQ, which is also designed for patients seen in the primary care setting[11] and is the most recently developed and validated PRO measure.[12] This instrument has 6 questions (**Table 2**).[13] The basis for this PRO is the data gathered from the Diamond study. The GERDQ questions are derived from the RDQ, the Gastrointestinal Symptom Rating Scale (GSRS), and the Gastroesophageal Reflux Disease Impact Scale (GIS).[11]

In patients with a GERDQ total score of 8 or more, approximately 80% have GERD and, in those with a total score between 3 and 7, 50% have GERD. None with a score of 0 to 2 had GERD.[11] Of these cutoffs, a total GERDQ score of 8 has the highest specificity (71.4%) and sensitivity (64.6%) and is the optimal cutoff proposed for the diagnosis of GERD, reaching a diagnostic accuracy similar to that of a gastroenterologist. In contrast, a total score of 2 or less suggests a very low likelihood of GERD.[11]

Two recent studies comparing a structured approach based on the GERDQ scores with a traditional approach showed the significant advantages of identifying and treating patients with a high likelihood of having GERD without further testing. These advantages are measured in terms of clinical outcomes and reduced costs.[14,15] In 2011, Lacy and colleagues[16] reported on 358 consecutive patients (180 were off proton pump inhibitors [PPIs]) referred to them from both primary care providers and specialists, with symptoms thought to be secondary to GERD for a 48-hour esophageal wireless pH study. In this patient population, the investigators concluded that the GERDQ (with a cutoff total score of ≥8) has only modest sensitivity (71% in patients

---

Table 1
RDQ items and scoring system used by Kahrilas and colleagues

Reflux Disease Questionnaire (RDQ)

*Please answer each question by ticking **one** box per row*

1. **Thinking about your symptoms over the past 7 days, how often did you have the following?**

	Did not have	Less than 1 day a week	1 day a week	2-3 days a week	4-6 days a week	Daily
a. A burning feeling behind your breastbone	☐	☐	☐	☐	☐	☐
b. Pain behind your breastbone	☐	☐	☐	☐	☐	☐
c. A burning feeling in the centre of the upper stomach	☐	☐	☐	☐	☐	☐
d. A pain in the centre of the upper stomach	☐	☐	☐	☐	☐	☐
e. An acid taste in your mouth	☐	☐	☐	☐	☐	☐
f. Unpleasant movement of material upwards from the stomach	☐	☐	☐	☐	☐	☐

2. **Thinking about your symptoms over the past 7 days, how would you rate the following?**

	Did not have	Very mild	Mild	Moderate	Moderately severe	Severe
a. A burning feeling behind your breastbone	☐	☐	☐	☐	☐	☐
b. Pain behind your breastbone	☐	☐	☐	☐	☐	☐
c. A burning feeling in the centre of the upper stomach	☐	☐	☐	☐	☐	☐
d. A pain in the centre of the upper stomach	☐	☐	☐	☐	☐	☐
e. An acid taste in your mouth	☐	☐	☐	☐	☐	☐
f. Unpleasant movement of material upwards from the stomach	☐	☐	☐	☐	☐	☐

From Kahrilas PJ, Jonsson A, Denison H, et al. Regurgitation is less responsive to acid suppression than heartburn in patients with gastroesophageal reflux disease. Clin Gastroenterol Hepatol 2012;10(6):612–9; with permission.

off PPI and 55% on PPI) and specificity (41% in patients off PPI and 52% on PPI) using abnormal acid exposure as the basis for diagnosis. In a letter to the editor, Vakil and Kahrilas[17] stated that GERDQ was not designed for patients referred for wireless pH testing because this group of patients comprise a selected group of patients with symptoms refractory to therapy. In response, Lacy and colleagues[18] stated that even though questionnaires to diagnose acid reflux have distinct advantages (ie, ease of use, cost, and safety), the investigators were not convinced that current

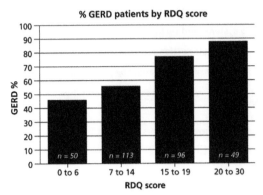

Fig. 3. Proposed management algorithm in primary care. (*From* Dent J, Vakil N, Jones R, et al. Accuracy of the diagnosis of GORD by questionnaire, physicians and a trial of proton pump inhibitor treatment: the Diamond Study. Gut 2010;59(6):714–21; with permission.)

questionnaires are effective, and proposed that large, multinational, prospective trials comparing validated questionnaires with endoscopy and pH monitoring are needed. Therefore use of the GERDQ in a gastroenterology/subspecialty practice may not be practical or beneficial.

SENSITIVITY AND SPECIFICITY FOR HEARTBURN IN DIAGNOSING GERD
Estimated Range Based on Recent Reviews

pH monitoring of patients with heartburn as the predominant symptom (specialty practice) has a sensitivity of 78% and specificity of 68%. Based on empiric PPI therapy in patients with heartburn as the predominant symptom (primary care), the estimated sensitivity ranges from 70% to 80%, with specificity of 55% to 65%.[4]

Table 2
GERDQ self-assessment questionnaire used by Tielemans and colleagues

Symptoms in the Previous Week	Symptom Presence			
Question:	0 d	1 d	2–3 d	4–7 d
1 How often did you have a burning feeling behind your breastbone (heartburn)?	0	1	2	3
2 How often did you have stomach contents (liquid or food) moving upwards to your throat or mouth (regurgitation)?	0	1	2	3
3 How often did you have a pain in the center of the upper stomach?	3	2	1	0
4 How often did you have nausea?	3	2	1	0
5 How often did you have difficulty getting a good night's sleep because of your heartburn and/or regurgitation?	0	1	2	3
6 How often did you take additional medication for your heartburn and/or regurgitation other than what the physician told you to take (such as Maalox)?	0	1	2	3

From Tielemans MM, van Oijen MG. Online follow-up of individuals with gastroesophageal reflux disease using a patient-reported outcomes instrument: results of an observational study. BMC Gastroenterol 2013;13(1):144.

A systematic review by Moayyedi and colleagues[19] reported a sensitivity of heartburn and regurgitation of 30% to 76% for the presence of erosive esophagitis, with specificity from 62% to 96%.

Based on data from the Diamond study, the presence of heartburn or regurgitation as the most troublesome symptom gives an overall sensitivity of 49% with a specificity of 74%. If either heartburn or regurgitation is the most or second most troublesome symptom, the sensitivity is increased to 69%, accompanied by an expected decrease in specificity to 62%.[10]

These are probably the best estimates of specificity and sensitivity available for the symptoms of heartburn and regurgitation. The sensitivities/specificities for diagnosis of GERD were marginally higher among gastroenterologists at 67%/70% versus family practitioners at 63%/63%.

DIFFICULTY WITH USING HEARTBURN AS THE PRIMARY MEANS OF DIAGNOSING GERD: COMMON OCCURRENCE OF HEARTBURN WITH OTHER SYMPTOMS

Heartburn symptoms rarely occur without other symptoms, such as dyspepsia.[20] This association indicates that heartburn and regurgitation occur frequently in patients with functional dyspepsia, even after objective GERD has been exhaustively excluded by appropriate testing. In an accompanying editorial, Talley[21] proposes that functional dyspepsia and heartburn may have the same mechanisms. Based on a systematic literature review conducted in patients with GERD, dyspeptic symptoms (epigastric pain, bloating, early satiety, nausea, and vomiting) were present in 38% $\pm$ 14% of patients with GERD and occurred more frequently in patients with GERD with more frequent symptoms compared with patients with intermittent or no GERD symptoms.[22] Based on the Diamond study, dyspepsia is as common among patients with GERD as it is in patients without GERD as the most troublesome symptom (GERD, 21.2%; non-GERD, 22.9%) or second most troublesome symptom (GERD, 17.2%; non-GERD, 19%).[10]

SENSITIVITY AND SPECIFICITY OF REGURGITATION IN DIAGNOSING GERD

The sensitivity and specificity of regurgitation are difficult to determine independently of heartburn. In the same group of patients mentioned earlier who were referred for a pH study, the positive predictive value of heartburn increased from 59% to 66% when regurgitation was also present.[4]

PPI USE IN GERD

PPI is the most effective pharmacologic treatment of patients with traditionally defined GERD; that is, patients with heartburn and an abnormal endoscopy (reflux esophagitis). Based on a Cochrane Review by Khan and colleagues,[23] the number needed to treat to have benefit (NNTB) for healing of esophagitis is 1.7. In contrast, the NNTB for complete heartburn control among a group of patients with negative endoscopy reflux disease (NERD) as entry criteria is 3 to 4.[24] The pooled response rate at 4 weeks of NERD versus erosive esophagitis (RE) patients is 37% versus 56%. In contrast, a 2012 meta-analysis by Weijenborg and colleagues[25] inferred that, in a well-defined group of patients with NERD (negative endoscopy and a positive pH test) the estimated complete symptom response rate after PPI therapy was comparable with patients with RE. The pooled estimate of complete relief of heartburn after 4 weeks of PPI therapy in patients with narrowly defined (endoscopy negative/positive pH test) NERD is 0.73 (95% confidence interval [CI], 0.69–0.77 from 2 studies). In patients with RE this was calculated at 0.72 (95% CI, 0.69–0.74 from 32 studies) versus NERD defined as negative endoscopy alone with a pooled estimate of complete relief of 0.49 (95% CI, 0.44–0.55 from 12 studies).[25]

THE PPI TEST

One of the most difficult aspects of using the PPI test is the lack of consensus for key components defining the test: the particular PPI, the PPI dosage and time of administration (single dose vs double dose, once a day vs twice a day), the duration of treatment (7, 14, or 28 days), the definition of treatment response (complete relief of symptoms vs proportion of symptom relief). As early as 1995 the PPI test was administered to patients with erosive esophagitis and nonerosive esophagitis.[26] de Leone and colleagues[27] recently enrolled 544 patients undergoing an upper endoscopy for heartburn (with or without regurgitation) for 15 days, at least once a day for the previous 3 months before enrollment. In this study, the diagnosis of GERD was not confirmed by a pH study. Based on these data and the ROC curves for different thresholds and durations, the investigators inferred that the ideal PPI test would be a twice-daily regimen lasting for 1 week with at least a 75% reduction in heartburn symptoms (with or without regurgitation). The PPI test response in this study was higher than has been previously reported.

In 2004, Numans and colleagues[28] published a meta-analysis about the PPI test for GERD diagnosis. The investigators included 15 studies that compared clinical response with a short course of a PPI with an objective measure of GERD, such as 24-hour pH monitoring. Combined estimates with 24-hour pH monitoring as the reference standard yielded a value for sensitivity of 0.78 (95% CI, 0.66–0.86) and for specificity of 0.54 (95% CI, 0.44–0.65). These values were lower when endoscopy results and symptom scores were used as the reference standards. The investigators concluded that the PPI test for patients suspected of having GERD does not confidently establish or exclude the diagnosis of GERD, defined by the presence of RE or a positive pH test. Bytzer and colleagues[29] recently analyzed the results of the Diamond study and noted that there was a positive PPI test in 69% of patients with GERD (confirmed by pH and/or esophagitis on endoscopy) compared with 51% of patients without GERD. The investigators concluded that the PPI test is not a definitive test for GERD because of the significant proportion of patients without GERD showing a positive result for the PPI test. Moreover, the use of the total RDQ score in the Diamond study together with the PPI test added little value, because response to the PPI test did not correlate with the baseline RDQ score.[10] There is a benefit to obtaining the RDQ score: based on a cutoff RDQ score of greater than 15, patients with GERD with typical symptoms (heartburn, regurgitation central chest pain, and dysphagia) had a greater proportion of responders (69%) versus patients with atypical (dyspepsia) symptoms (38%).[10]

In terms of duration of the PPI test, based on the work of de Leone and colleagues[27] and Bytzer and colleagues,[29] the response to the PPI plateaus at day 7 of therapy (Fig. 4).

The PPI test does not have the performance characteristics of an acceptable diagnostic test to establish or exclude a diagnosis of GERD. However, using the PPI test makes sense from a cost-effectiveness and usefulness standpoint. In an editorial, van Zanten[30] notes that even though this test may not be specific enough to exclude non-GERD–related diagnoses, the patient's positive response to a PPI resulting in complete relief of upper gastrointestinal symptoms (be they peptic ulcer disease or GERD) is still a positive response and of benefit for the patient.[30]

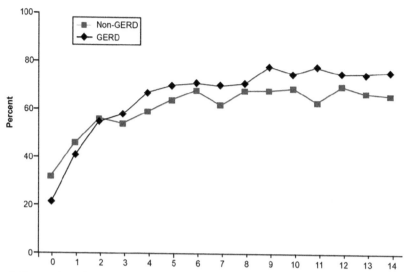

Fig. 4. Proportion of patients with relief of reflux symptoms in response to PPI day by day. (*From* Bytzer P, Jones R, Vakil N, et al. Limited ability of the proton-pump inhibitor test to identify patients with gastroesophageal reflux disease. Clin Gastroenterol Hepatol 2012;10(12):1360–6; with permission.)

Using the GERDQ as the initial screening tool in a clinical pathway approach for the diagnosis of typical symptoms of GERD is a reasonable alternative (**Fig. 5**).[31] Again, the important score intervals are a cutoff value of 8 or more, which has the highest specificity and sensitivity; a total score of 3 to 7, which is less sensitive (50% positive

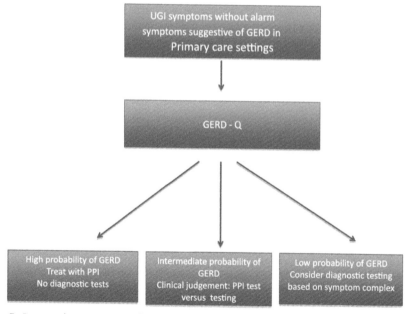

Fig. 5. Proposed management algorithm in primary care. (*From* Vakil N. The initial diagnosis of GERD. Best Pract Res Clin Gastroenterol 2013;27(3):365–71; with permission.)

for a diagnosis of GERD); and, in those with a score of 2 or less, no patients were diagnosed to have GERD. No questionnaire is applicable to patients with alarm characteristics (ie, dysphagia, weight loss, anemia, long-standing symptoms, and a family history of adenocarcinoma of the esophagus).

The PPI test for the diagnosis of GERD at this point may be best defined as:

1. A total dosage of 40 mg of omeprazole (or equivalent dosage of another PPI) once a day or the use of 20 mg of omeprazole (or equivalent dosage of another PPI) given twice a day
2. Treatment duration of 1 week
3. Treatment response measured as symptom reduction of at least 75%

In the primary care setting, the PPI test is best performed in conjunction with a PRO measure (RDQ or GERDQ) documenting that the patient has typical symptoms (heartburn with or without regurgitation) that are both frequent and severe.

REGURGITATION AND ACID SUPPRESSION

In a systematic review reporting on the response of regurgitation to PPI therapy, Kahrilas and colleagues[32] noted that regurgitation was neither an entry requirement nor the primary end point in any of the 31 clinical trials they identified. Owing to the variability in the definition of regurgitation and the primary use of investigator-reported assessment in more than half of these trials, no meta-analysis was attempted. Based on analysis of data from 2 randomized control trials of AZD0865 versus esomeprazole for the treatment of NERD versus RE, Kahrilas and colleagues[32] concluded that regurgitation was less responsive to acid suppression than heartburn in patients with GERD, indicating that persistent regurgitation is a common cause of incomplete treatment response.

In summary, neither the symptom of heartburn (with or without regurgitation) nor the PPI test has the test characteristics to diagnose or exclude GERD as a diagnosis. There are sufficient data to support the use of PROs (RDQ or GERDQ) as a part of a clinical pathway in primary care to capture disease severity in conjunction with the PPI test.

REFERENCES

1. Spechler SJ, Jain SK, Tendler DA, et al. Racial differences in the frequency of symptoms and complications of gastro-oesophageal reflux disease. Aliment Pharmacol Ther 2002;16(10):1795–800.
2. Sharma P, Wani S, Romero Y, et al. Racial and geographic issues in gastroesophageal reflux disease. Am J Gastroenterol 2008;103(11):2669–80.
3. Lacy BE, Weiser K, Chertoff J, et al. The diagnosis of gastroesophageal reflux disease. Am J Med 2010;123(7):583–92.
4. Kuo P, Holloway RH. A pragmatic symptom-based approach. Best Pract Res Clin Gastroenterol 2010;24(6):765–73.
5. Lin M, Gerson LB, Lascar R, et al. Features of gastroesophageal reflux disease in women. Am J Gastroenterol 2004;99(8):1442–7.
6. McColl E, Junghard O, Wiklund I, et al. Assessing symptoms in gastroesophageal reflux disease: how well do clinicians' assessments agree with those of their patients? Am J Gastroenterol 2005;100(1):11–8.
7. Dent J. Review article: towards the optimization of symptom evaluation in reflux disease. Aliment Pharmacol Ther 2004;20(Suppl 5):14–8 [discussion: 38–9].

8. Chassany O, Shaheen NJ, Karlsson M, et al. Systematic review: symptom assessment using patient-reported outcomes in gastroesophageal reflux disease and dyspepsia. Scand J Gastroenterol 2012;47(12):1412–21.
9. Vakil NB, Halling K, Becher A, et al. Systematic review of patient-reported outcome instruments for gastroesophageal reflux disease symptoms. Eur J Gastroenterol Hepatol 2013;25(1):2–14.
10. Dent J, Vakil N, Jones R, et al. Accuracy of the diagnosis of GORD by questionnaire, physicians and a trial of proton pump inhibitor treatment: the Diamond Study. Gut 2010;59(6):714–21.
11. Jones R, Junghard O, Dent J, et al. Development of the GerdQ, a tool for the diagnosis and management of gastro-oesophageal reflux disease in primary care. Aliment Pharmacol Ther 2009;30(10):1030–8.
12. Jonasson C, Wernersson B, Hoff DA, et al. Validation of the GerdQ questionnaire for the diagnosis of gastro-oesophageal reflux disease. Aliment Pharmacol Ther 2013;37(5):564–72.
13. Tielemans MM, van Oijen MG. Online follow-up of individuals with gastroesophageal reflux disease using a patient-reported outcomes instrument: results of an observational study. BMC Gastroenterol 2013;13(1):144.
14. Jonasson C, Moum B, Bang C, et al. Randomised clinical trial: a comparison between a GerdQ-based algorithm and an endoscopy-based approach for the diagnosis and initial treatment of GERD. Aliment Pharmacol Ther 2012;35(11):1290–300.
15. Bergquist H, Agreus L, Tillander L, et al. Structured diagnostic and treatment approach versus the usual primary care approach in patients with gastroesophageal reflux disease: a cluster-randomized multicenter study. J Clin Gastroenterol 2013;47(7):e65–73.
16. Lacy BE, Chehade R, Crowell MD. A prospective study to compare a symptom-based reflux disease questionnaire to 48-h wireless pH monitoring for the identification of gastroesophageal reflux (revised 2-26-11). Am J Gastroenterol 2011; 106(9):1604–11.
17. Vakil N, Kahrilas PJ. GERD diagnosis: pretest probability and the "gold" standard alter outcome. Am J Gastroenterol 2012;107(2):322–3 [author reply: 323–4].
18. Lacy BE, Chehade R, Crowell MD. Response to Vakil and Kahrilas. Am J Gastroenterol 2012;107(2):323–4.
19. Moayyedi P, Talley NJ, Fennerty MB, et al. Can the clinical history distinguish between organic and functional dyspepsia? JAMA 2006;295(13):1566–76.
20. Vakil N, Halling K, Ohlsson L, et al. Symptom overlap between postprandial distress and epigastric pain syndromes of the Rome III dyspepsia classification. Am J Gastroenterol 2013;108(5):767–74.
21. Talley NJ. Functional (non-ulcer) dyspepsia and gastroesophageal reflux disease: one not two diseases? Am J Gastroenterol 2013;108(5):775–7.
22. Gerson LB, Kahrilas PJ, Fass R. Insights into gastroesophageal reflux disease-associated dyspeptic symptoms. Clin Gastroenterol Hepatol 2011;9(10):824–33.
23. Khan M, Santana J, Donnellan C, et al. Medical treatments in the short term management of reflux oesophagitis. Cochrane Database Syst Rev 2007;(2):CD003244.
24. Dean BB, Gano AD Jr, Knight K, et al. Effectiveness of proton pump inhibitors in nonerosive reflux disease. Clin Gastroenterol Hepatol 2004;2(8):656–64.
25. Weijenborg PW, Cremonini F, Smout AJ, et al. PPI therapy is equally effective in well-defined non-erosive reflux disease and in reflux esophagitis: a meta-analysis. Neurogastroenterol Motil 2012;24(8):747–57 e350.
26. Schindlbeck NE, Klauser AG, Voderholzer WA, et al. Empiric therapy for gastroesophageal reflux disease. Arch Intern Med 1995;155(16):1808–12.

27. de Leone A, Tonini M, Dominici P, et al. The proton pump inhibitor test for gastro-esophageal reflux disease: optimal cut-off value and duration. Dig Liver Dis 2010; 42(11):785–90.
28. Numans ME, Lau J, de Wit NJ, et al. Short-term treatment with proton-pump inhibitors as a test for gastroesophageal reflux disease: a meta-analysis of diagnostic test characteristics. Ann Intern Med 2004;140(7):518–27.
29. Bytzer P, Jones R, Vakil N, et al. Limited ability of the proton-pump inhibitor test to identify patients with gastroesophageal reflux disease. Clin Gastroenterol Hepatol 2012;10(12):1360–6.
30. Veldhuyzen van Zanten S. Diamond GERD diagnosis studies: clinical feelings are good, but are measurements using a PPI test better? Clin Gastroenterol Hepatol 2012;10(12):1367–8.
31. Vakil N. The initial diagnosis of GERD. Best Pract Res Clin Gastroenterol 2013; 27(3):365–71.
32. Kahrilas PJ, Jonsson A, Denison H, et al. Regurgitation is less responsive to acid suppression than heartburn in patients with gastroesophageal reflux disease. Clin Gastroenterol Hepatol 2012;10(6):612–9.

Role of Endoscopy in GERD

Virender K. Sharma, MD

KEYWORDS

- Endoscopy • GERD • Barrett • Diagnosis • Therapy • Esophagitis

KEY POINTS

- Endoscopy is the mainstay diagnostic and therapeutic tool in the management of GERD.
- Endoscopy is recommended for the evaluation of medically refractory or atypical GERD, patients with alarm symptoms of dysphagia, anemia or weight loss, for diagnosis and surveillance of Barrett esophagus in patients with chronic GERD, and for application of such therapies as esophageal dilation or ablation.
- Newer imaging techniques in development will further improve the accuracy and use of endoscopy in management of GERD.

INTRODUCTION

Gastroesophageal reflux disease (GERD) is one of the most common conditions encountered in primary care and gastroenterology practices. Almost 40% of the US population suffers from occasional heartburn and up to 20% of patients report bothersome symptoms on at least a weekly basis. Heartburn or indigestion is the commonest symptom of GERD and accounts for nearly 2 million outpatient clinic visits, with dysphagia accounting for additional 1 million visits. GERD is the leading diagnosis for gastrointestinal disorders in outpatient clinic visits in the United States accounting for almost 9 million visits in the year 2009, with Barrett esophagus accounting for an additional 500,000 visits. Endoscopy is commonly performed for the diagnosis and management of GERD, with reflux symptoms (24%) and dysphagia (20%) being the commonest indications.[1]

The prevalence of GERD and use of endoscopy for management of GERD are rising. In a systemic analysis, El-Serag[2] reported an increasing prevalence of GERD over the last two decades. Analysis of CORI and CMMS databases shows an increased use of endoscopy partially accounted for by rising prevalence of GERD.[3]

This article discusses the appropriate indications for endoscopy in patients with GERD and highlights newer imaging technologies that may improve utility and outcomes of endoscopy in management of GERD.

Disclosure Statement: Consultant Takeda Pharmaceuticals, Equity/Consultant EndoStim Inc.
Arizona Digestive Health, 2680 South Val Vista, Suite 116, Gilbert, AZ 85295, USA
E-mail address: vksharma@arizonadigestivehealth.com

Gastroenterol Clin N Am 43 (2014) 39–46
http://dx.doi.org/10.1016/j.gtc.2013.12.003
0889-8553/14/$ – see front matter © 2014 Elsevier Inc. All rights reserved.

ESOPHAGOGASTRODUODENOSCOPY OR UPPER ENDOSCOPY

High-definition, high-resolution flexible video endoscopy has become the standard of endoscopic care in the United States. Esophagogastroduodenoscopy allows for excellent view of the mucosal details and allows for obtaining photographs, video recordings, and tissue sampling using biopsy and brush cytology. Endoscopy also allows for application of therapies, such as esophageal dilation, Barrett ablation, and endoscopic resection of preneoplastic and early neoplastic lesions. Most esophago-gastroduodenoscopy procedures in the United States are performed using conscious sedation or procedural sedations. However, data suggest that unsedated, thin-scope esophagogastroduodenoscopy can be safely and successfully performed in carefully selected patients.[4]

Advances in imaging technology are expanding the accuracy of traditional white light endoscopy. High-definition (>850,000 pixel density), high-magnification (>115×) endoscopes using 1080p technology allow one to see mucosal details with greater resolution improving its diagnostic accuracy. Electronic or virtual chromoendoscopy is replacing traditional chromoendoscopy using dye, which was cumbersome and messy.

Standard white light endoscopy uses blue, green, and red light waves, whereas the NBI technology (Olympus, Center Valley, PA), using electronic light filters, only uses blue (440–460 nm) and green (540–560 nm) wave light, eliminating the use of the red light. The narrower wavelengths highlight the superficial mucosa and blood vessels accentuating the mucosal architecture and microvasculature. The FICE system (Fuji, Wayne, NJ) and I-Scan (Pentax, Montvale, NJ) use postprocessing techniques, such as spectral analysis, or postprocessing enhancements to achieve electronic chromoendoscopy.

Full-spectrum endoscopy (FUSE; EndoChoice, Atlanta, GA) allows for a 245-degree field of view compared with the 160-degree field of view of traditional upper endoscopy and may improve the diagnostic yield of upper endoscopy.

CONFOCAL LASER ENDOMICROSCOPY AND OPTICAL COHERENCE TOMOGRAPHY

Confocal laser endomicroscopy and optical coherence tomography (OCT) use lasers to penetrate to a certain depth below the surface and magnify the images obtained to evaluate deeper structures. Two catheter-based technologies for confocal laser endomicroscopy (Cellvizio; Mauna Kea Technologies, Paris, France) and OCT (NvisionVLE; Ninepoint Medical, Cambridge, MA) have been approved by the Food and Drug Administration for use in the United States.

The Cellvizio probe-based confocal laser endomicroscopy system uses a 7F catheter confocal miniprobe, which is passed down the working channel of the upper endoscope and a low-power blue laser light (wave length 488 nm) passed through a fiberoptic bundle for tissue illumination after application of fluorescence agents (topical Acriflavine hydrochloride and Cresyl Violet, and systemic fluorescein) to obtain confocal images (~1000 × magnification) of the mucosa fixed image plane depth of 55 to 65 μm that are streamed at a frame rate of 12 frames per second.

OCT uses a technique called interferometry that measures the path length of reflected light and processes the information for image generation, a technique similar to an ultrasound that uses sound waves. The NvisionVLE OCT or volumetric laser endomicroscopy uses a balloon catheter that passes through a 2.8-mm or larger scope channel and performs volumetric laser interferometry based on frequency domain OCT to faster, real-time, high-resolution imaging. It provides resolution to 10 mm and imaging depth down to 3 mm, real-time resolution of 7 μm, scanning over a 6-cm length of esophagus for a period of 90 seconds and allowing for the visualization of tissue layers including the esophageal mucosa, submucosa, and muscularis propria.

WIRELESS CAPSULE ENDOSCOPY

Esophageal capsule endoscopy was approved by the Food and Drug Administration in 2004 for the evaluation of the esophagus in patients with GERD and suspected Barrett esophagus. Esophageal capsule endoscopy uses a video capsule endoscope with camera at both ends (height, 11 mm; width, 26 mm; weight, 3.7 g) that takes images of the esophagus at 18 frames per seconds. Esophageal capsule endoscopy allowed for unsedated outpatient evaluation of the esophagus with moderate sensitivity and specificity for the evaluation of Barrett esophagus.[5] However, because of cost and need for mucosal biopsy for the diagnosis of Barrett esophagus, it is not widely used. A tethered multiuse string capsule using the small bowel capsule endoscope was developed to overcome some of the issues of traditional esophageal capsule endoscopy but interest in the technology has waned.[6]

GASTROESOPHAGEAL REFLUX DISEASE

Montreal Consensus Conference defines GERD as a condition that develops when there is reflux of stomach contents into the esophagus causing troublesome symptoms, complications, or both.[7] Presence of mucosal damage and positive endoscopic findings are not a prerequisite for the diagnosis of GERD. GERD can accurately be diagnosed by history of classical symptoms of heartburn and/or regurgitation and a positive response to antisecretory therapy.[7] Almost two-thirds of patients with GERD have nonerosive disease and a normal endoscopy.[8] Los Angeles classification (**Table 1**) is most commonly used to classify the grade of erosive esophagitis in the United States, whereas the Savary-Miller classification is more commonly used in Europe. Los Angeles classification has been shown to have good intraobserver and interobserver agreement among experienced and inexperienced endoscopists and correlates well with the amount of esophageal acid exposure and complications of GERD.[9] However, neither of the classifications accurately predicts symptom severity.

The Clinical Guidelines Committee of the American College of Physicians recommends endoscopy in (1) patients with heartburn and alarm symptoms (dysphagia, bleeding, anemia, weight loss, and recurrent vomiting), (2) typical GERD symptoms that persist despite a therapeutic trial of 4 to 8 weeks of twice-daily proton-pump inhibitor therapy, (3) patients with severe (greater than or equal to Los Angeles grade

Table 1	
Los Angeles classification of endoscopic grades of esophagitis	
Grade	**Endoscopic Description**
A	One or more mucosal break <5 mm that does not extend between the tops of two mucosal folds
B	One or more mucosal break ≥5 mm that does not extend between the tops of two mucosal folds
C	One or more mucosal break that is continuous between the tops of two or more mucosal folds but that involves <75% of the circumference
D	One or more mucosal break that involves ≥75% of the esophageal circumference

C-D) erosive esophagitis after a 2-month course of proton-pump inhibitor therapy to assess healing and rule out Barrett esophagus, and (4) history of esophageal stricture who have recurrent symptoms of dysphagia.[3]

In addition to the above indications, the American Society for Gastrointestinal Endoscopy recommends endoscopy in patients with either extraesophageal symptoms or atypical symptoms of GERD. Endoscopy should also be performed as a part of preoperative evaluation and for the evaluation of patients with recurrent symptoms after endoscopic or surgical antireflux procedures.[10] The American College of Gastroenterology recommends endoscopy to diagnose complications of GERD and identify suspected Barrett esophagus in patients with chronic GERD.[11] Although the American Gastroenterological Association recommends endoscopy for patients with chronic GERD with troublesome dysphagia and nonresponsive to empiric trial of twice-daily proton-pump inhibitor, alarm symptoms other than troublesome dysphagia are classified as "insufficient evidence" to make a recommendation. Biopsies of esophageal abnormalities are recommended; however, routine biopsy of normal squamous mucosa for the diagnosis of GERD is not recommended. Esophageal biopsies (at least five samples) should be performed if the differential diagnosis of eosinophilic esophagitis is being considered (**Box 1**).[12]

ESOPHAGEAL DILATION

Esophageal stricture formation is a well-known complication of GERD. However, the incidence of recurrent stricture has decreased with widespread use of antisecretory therapy with proton-pump inhibitors. Dysphagia is the primary indication for endoscopic dilation and need for dilation in the absence of dysphagia or empiric dilation for dysphagia in the absence of structural abnormality is not routinely recommended.[13]

Three types of dilators are routinely used to perform endoscopic dilation: (1) non–wire-guided mercury or tungsten-filled bougies (Maloney or Hurst), (2) wire-guided polyvinyl dilators (Savary- Gilliard or American), and (3) through-the-scope balloon dilators. Maloney dilators are passed blindly and may have higher risk of perforation compared with wire-guided Savary dilators or through-the-scope balloon dilators. Use of fluoroscopy with Maloney dilators is advised for improved safety and functional results. To avoid complications with dilation, a conservative approach to dilation is the "rule of three," which recommends that after moderate resistance is encountered with

---

Box 1
Indications for endoscopy in GERD

Persistent or progressive GERD symptoms despite appropriate medical therapy

Atypical GERD symptoms

Evaluation of patients with suspected extraesophageal manifestations of GERD

Alarm symptoms

 Dysphagia or odynophagia

 Involuntary weight loss, evidence of gastrointestinal bleeding, or anemia

 Finding of a mass, stricture, or ulcer on imaging studies

Screening for Barrett esophagus in selected patients (as clinically indicated)

Evaluation of patients' before and with recurrent symptoms after endoscopic or surgical antireflux procedures

the bougie dilator, no greater than three consecutive dilators in increments of 1 mm should be used in a single dilation session. In patients with dysphagia caused by Schatzki ring, a larger 16- to 20-mm dilator should be used with the intent of disrupting the stricture.[13] Biopsy of the Schatzki ring before dilation may help in effectively breaking the ring with dilation.

BARRETT ESOPHAGUS

Barrett esophagus is a metaplastic change of the esophageal lining from the normal squamous to specialized columnar epithelium caused by chronic acid damage. Approximately 10% of patients with chronic heartburn symptoms have Barrett esophagus accounting for almost a half million of the visits in 2009.[1] An estimated 3.3 million Americans have a diagnosis of Barrett esophagus. White men have the highest risk for Barrett esophagus, with women, African-Americans, and Asians having lower risks. Hispanics have comparable prevalence of Barrett esophagus as whites.[14] Most (90%) patients with Barrett esophagus have nondysplastic disease and a very low rate of progression to esophageal adenocarcinoma at a rate of 0.3 to 0.4 per patient-year.[15] Guidelines generally recommend that patients with nondysplastic disease undergo endoscopic surveillance every 3 to 5 years to detect progression to dysplasia and/or esophageal adenocarcinoma. Given the large number of subjects with Barrett esophagus, these examinations represent a substantial commitment of resources.

Men older than 50 years with chronic GERD symptoms greater than 5-years duration, nocturnal reflux symptoms, hiatal hernia, elevated body mass index, tobacco use, intra-abdominal distribution of fat, and family history of esophageal cancer are at highest risk for Barrett esophagus and esophageal adenocarcinoma.[3]

The Clinical Guidelines Committee of the American College of Physicians recommends endoscopy in men older than 50 years with chronic (>5 years) GERD symptoms and additional risk factors (nocturnal reflux symptoms, hiatal hernia, elevated body mass index, tobacco use, and intra-abdominal distribution of fat) to detect esophageal adenocarcinoma and Barrett esophagus. In men and women with Barrett esophagus and no dysplasia, surveillance examinations should occur at intervals no more frequently than 3 to 5 years. More frequent intervals are indicated in patients with Barrett esophagus and dysplasia (**Box 2**).[3]

American College of Gastroenterology recommends endoscopy for diagnosis of Barrett esophagus in patients with chronic GERD symptoms. In patients with nondysplastic Barrett esophagus, the recommendation is repeat endoscopy at 1 year and

---

Box 2
Indications for endoscopy for Barrett esophagus

Men older than 50 years with chronic (>5 years) GERD symptoms for detection of Barrett esophagus

Every 3–5 years in patients with nondysplastic Barrett esophagus[a]

In 6 months to confirm the diagnosis of low-grade dysplasia and then annually[b]

Every 3 months in patients with high-grade dysplasia[b]

[a] American College of Gastroenterology guidelines recommend repeat endoscopy in 1 year to exclude incident dysplasia and cancer and then every 3 years; American Gastroenterological Association guidelines recommend endoscopy every 5 years.
[b] Consider endoscopic ablative therapy in select patients.

then 3-year intervals to monitor for progression to dysplasia. Patient with low-grade dysplasia should undergo surveillance at 6- to 12-month intervals and with high-grade dysplasia (HGD) at 3-month intervals. Definitive therapy in the form of ablation or surgery should be considered in patients with HGD.[11]

American Gastroenterological Association guidelines consider the evidence to be insufficient to recommend routine upper endoscopy in the setting of chronic GERD symptoms to diminish the risk of death from esophageal cancer and endoscopic screening for Barrett esophagus and dysplasia in adults 50 years or older with more than 5 to 10 years of heartburn to reduce mortality from esophageal adenocarcinoma.[12]

American Society for Gastrointestinal Endoscopy guidelines recommend endoscopic screening for Barrett esophagus in select patients with multiple risk factors for Barrett esophagus and esophageal adenocarcinoma with the caveat that the patient be informed that there is insufficient evidence to affirm this recommendation. Periodic endoscopic surveillance based on histologic grade and endoscopic ablative therapy in selected patients is recommended.[10]

ADVANCE IMAGING

A recent meta-analysis of electronic or virtual chromoendoscopy showed a 34% increased yield for the diagnosis of dysplasia in patients with Barrett esophagus and the increased yield was comparable with traditional chromoendoscopy without the added hassle or cost of using dyes. The authors recommended targeted biopsies using electronic chromoendoscopy followed by random biopsies using the Seattle protocol as being ideal for dysplasia detection.[16]

Two trials of probe-based confocal endomicroscopy have shown high negative predictive value of this technique, reducing the number of biopsies required and increasing assurance to patients with negative tests, thus overcoming the issue of sampling error and interobserver variability in biopsy interpretation in patients with Barrett esophagus undergoing surveillance.[17–19]

Preliminary results with volumetric laser endomicroscopy reveal a high accuracy in detecting HGD in patients with Barrett esophagus and also buried Barrett glands after ablative therapy.[20] Larger trials are awaited to conclusively establish the accuracy of this technique. However, generalizability of these advanced imaging techniques in accurate diagnosis outside expert academic institutions remains to be established.

EOSINOPHILIC ESOPHAGITIS

Eosinophilic esophagitis is increasingly recognized as a cause of esophageal symptoms, specifically solid food dysphagia and food impactions in the absence of typical GERD symptoms. However, many patients have overlap with both GERD and eosinophilic esophagitis. Additionally, patients with eosinophilic esophagitis can improve on acid suppression with proton-pump inhibitor therapy including patients with proton-pump inhibitor–responsive esophageal eosinophilia making the clinical diagnosis of eosinophilic esophagitis challenging. A high clinical suspicion and endoscopic findings of fixed esophageal rings (feline esophagus, trachealization, or corrugation), white exudates or plaques, longitudinal furrows, edema manifesting as mucosal pallor or decreased vascularity, diffuse esophageal narrowing, and mucosal fragility manifesting as esophageal lacerations induced by scope trauma are suggestive but not pathognomic of this disease. Esophageal biopsies (four to six samples) from mid and distal esophagus showing peak value of greater than or equal to 15 eosinophils per high-power field in the absence of other causes of mucosal eosinophilia are considered diagnostic of this condition.[21]

ENDOSCOPIC THERAPIES FOR GERD

There has been an ongoing attempt at the development of endoscopic therapies for the management of GERD. Most of these therapies were removed from practice because of lack of efficacy or because of safety concerns. There are currently two approved endoscopic GERD therapies available in the United States. Stretta (Mederi Therapeutics Inc, Greenwich, CT) radiofrequency therapy for GERD uses low-energy radiofrequency ablation of the submucosal tissue, resulting in increased lower esophageal sphincter compliance and decreased transient lower esophageal sphincter relaxation. Stretta therapy has been shown to improve esophageal pH and GERD symptoms and decrease medication use. Recently, Stretta therapy received a positive endorsement from the Society of American Gastrointestinal and Endoscopic Surgeons as being "appropriate therapy for patients being treated for GERD who are 18 years of age or older, who have had symptoms of heartburn, regurgitation, or both for 6 months or more, who have been partially or completely responsive to anti-secretory pharmacologic therapy, and who have declined laparoscopic fundoplication."[22]

Transoral fundoplication (EsophyX; EndoGastric Solution, Redwood City, WA) uses polypropylene H fasteners to create a serosa-to-serosa fusion to create a fundoplication. The results from multiple small open label studies reported a modest improvement in esophageal acid exposure, improvement in GERD symptoms, and reduction in medication usage. However, significant complications have been reported with this procedure and the Society of American Gastrointestinal and Endoscopic Surgeons issued a cautionary weak recommendation that transoral fundoplication may be an option for select patients. However, "more studies are needed to define optimal techniques and most appropriate patient selection criteria and to further evaluate device and technique safety."[22]

SUMMARY

Endoscopy is the most important diagnostic tool for evaluation and management of patients with GERD and Barrett esophagus. Newer imaging technologies hold promise in improving diagnostic accuracy. However, their validity and generalizability to routine clinical practice outside select academic institution need to be established.

REFERENCES

1. Peery AF, Dellon ES, LundBurden J, et al. Burden of gastrointestinal disease in the United States: 2012 update. Gastroenterology 2012;143:1179-87.
2. El-Serag HB. Time trends of gastroesophageal reflux disease: a systematic review. Clin Gastroenterol Hepatol 2007;5:17-26.
3. Shaheen NJ, Weinberg DS, Denberg TD, et al. Upper endoscopy for gastroesophageal reflux disease: best practice advice from the clinical guidelines committee of the American College of Physicians. Ann Intern Med 2012;157:808-16.
4. Peery AF, Hoppo T, Garman KS, et al. Feasibility, safety, acceptability, and yield of office-based, screening transnasal esophagoscopy. Gastrointest Endosc 2012; 75:945-53.
5. Eliakim R, Sharma VK, Yassin K, et al. A prospective study of the diagnostic accuracy of PillCam ESO esophageal capsule endoscopy versus conventional upper endoscopy in patients with chronic gastroesophageal reflux diseases. J Clin Gastroenterol 2005;39:572-8.

6. Ramirez FC, Akins R, Shaukat M. Screening of Barrett's esophagus with string-capsule endoscopy: a prospective blinded study of 100 consecutive patients using histology as the criterion standard. Gastrointest Endosc 2008;68:25–31.

7. Vakil N, van Zanten SV, Kahrilas P, et al. Global Consensus Group. The Montreal definition and classification of gastroesophageal reflux disease: a global evidence-based consensus. Am J Gastroenterol 2006;101:1900–20.

8. El-Serag HB. Epidemiology of non-erosive reflux disease. Digestion 2008; 78(Suppl 1):6–10.

9. Rath HC, Timmer A, Kunkel C, et al. Comparison of interobserver agreement for different scoring systems for reflux esophagitis: impact of level of experience. Gastrointest Endosc 2004;60:44–9.

10. Lichtenstein DR, Cash BD, Davila R, et al. Role of endoscopy in the management of GERD. Gastrointest Endosc 2007;66:219–24.

11. Katz PO, Gerson LB, Vela MF. Guidelines for the diagnosis and management of gastroesophageal reflux disease. Am J Gastroenterol 2013;108:308–28.

12. Kahrilas PJ, Shaheen NJ, Vaezi MF, et al. American Gastroenterological Association medical position statement on the management of gastroesophageal reflux disease. Gastroenterology 2008;135:1383–91.

13. Egan JV, Baron TH, Adler DA, et al. Esophageal dilation. Gastrointest Endosc 2006;63:755–60.

14. Balasubramanian G, Singh M, Gupta N, et al. Prevalence and predictors of columnar lined esophagus in gastroesophageal reflux disease (GERD) patients undergoing upper endoscopy. Am J Gastroenterol 2012;107:1655–61.

15. Lenglinger J, Riegler M, Cosentini E, et al. Review on the annual cancer risk of Barrett's esophagus in persons with symptoms of gastroesophageal reflux disease. Anticancer Res 2012;32:5465–73.

16. Qumseya BJ, Wang H, Badie N, et al. Advanced imaging technologies increase detection of dysplasia and neoplasia in patients with Barrett's esophagus: a meta-analysis and systematic review. Clin Gastroenterol Hepatol 2013;11: 1562–70.

17. Nguyen VX, Nguyen CC, De Petris G, et al. Confocal endomicroscopy (CEM) improves efficiency of Barrett surveillance. J Interv Gastroenterol 2012;2:61–5.

18. Sharma P, Meining AR, Coron E, et al. Real-time increased detection of neoplastic tissue in Barrett's esophagus with probe-based confocal laser endomicroscopy: final results of an international multicenter, prospective, randomized, controlled trial. Gastrointest Endosc 2011;74:465–72.

19. Bajbouj M, Vieth M, Rösch T, et al. Probe-based confocal laser endomicroscopy compared with standard four-quadrant biopsy for evaluation of neoplasia in Barrett's esophagus. Endoscopy 2010;42:435–40.

20. Leggett CL, Gorospe EC, Owens VL, et al. Can volumetric LASER endomicroscopy detect dysplasia in Barrett's esophagus? Gastrointest Endosc 2013;77: AB327.

21. Dellon ES, Gonsalves N, Hirano I, et al. ACG Clinical Guideline: evidenced based approach to the diagnosis and management of esophageal eosinophilia and eosinophilic esophagitis (EoE). Am J Gastroenterol 2013;108:679–92.

22. Auyang ED, Carter P, Rauth T, et al. SAGES Guidelines Committee. SAGES clinical spotlight review: endoluminal treatments for gastroesophageal reflux disease (GERD). Surg Endosc 2013;27:2658–72.

Barium Esophagram
Does It Have a Role in Gastroesophageal Reflux Disease?

Mark E. Baker, MD, FARS, FSCBT/MR[a,b,c,d,*],
David M. Einstein, MD, FARS[a,b]

KEYWORDS

- Barium esophagogram • Gastroesophageal reflux disease
- Post-fundoplication barium appearance

KEY POINTS

- The barium esophagram is an integral part of the assessment and management of patients with gastroesophageal reflux disease (GERD) before, and especially after, antireflux procedures.
- While many of the findings on the examination can be identified with endosocopy, a gastric emptying study and an esophageal motility examination, the barium esophagram is better at demonstrating the anatomic findings after antireflux surgery, especially in symptomatic patients.
- These complementary examinations, when taken as a whole, fully evaluate a patient with suspected GERD as well as symptomatic patients after antireflux procedures.

In the age of endoscopy, pH studies, and high-resolution manometry and impedance, the barium esophagram has been deemphasized in the diagnosis and management of patients with suspected gastroesophageal reflux disease (GERD). Unfortunately, as a result, as in most luminal gastrointestinal radiology, training for this important examination has suffered, resulting in the inability of recently trained radiologists to perform an adequate examination. Nevertheless, this examination is a vital part of a patient's workup when GERD is suspected.[1–4] This examination helps define both the morphology and function of the esophagus, identifying important findings relevant to treatment as well as suggesting diagnoses other than GERD. The authors believe that the examination is essential in defining the anatomic causes of symptoms after

[a] Cleveland Clinic Lerner College of Medicine, Case Western Reserve University, 9500 Euclid Avenue, Cleveland, OH 44195, USA; [b] Abdominal Imaging, Imaging Institute, Cleveland Clinic, 9500 Euclid Avenue, Cleveland, OH 44195, USA; [c] Digestive Disease Institute, Cleveland Clinic, 9500 Euclid Avenue, Cleveland, OH 44195, USA; [d] Cancer Institute, Cleveland Clinic, 9500 Euclid Avenue, Cleveland, OH 44195, USA
* Corresponding author. Abdominal Imaging, Imaging Institute, Cleveland Clinic, 9500 Euclid Avenue, Cleveland, OH 44195.
E-mail address: bakerm@ccf.org

Gastroenterol Clin N Am 43 (2014) 47–68
http://dx.doi.org/10.1016/j.gtc.2013.11.008
0889-8553/14/$ – see front matter © 2014 Elsevier Inc. All rights reserved.
gastro.theclinics.com

antireflux surgery. At the Cleveland Clinic many, if not most patients with suspected GERD are evaluated with a barium esophagram, especially if antireflux surgery is contemplated. Furthermore, all symptomatic patients after antireflux procedures are also evaluated with a barium esophagram.

ESOPHAGRAM: IMPORTANT GENERAL ELEMENTS OF THE EXAMINATION

Several factors are important to the success of a well-performed barium esophagram. First, the complete examination should be recorded in some fashion. A DVD recorder directly set up to the fluoroscopy unit will burn a DVD of the examination. With modern PACS (picture archiving and communication system), it is now possible to capture the fluoroscopic examination directly in DICOM (digital imaging and communications in medicine) format, and save the study without the hard-copy problems of a disk. Second, to reduce radiation exposure a pulsed-fluoroscopy unit is best, generally at 15 pulses per second, to reduce frame flickering. Third, if the patient has a specific complaint, such as dysphagia, before the start of the examination, the radiologist should encourage the patient to voice these symptoms when they occur during the examination.

Just before the examination, a brief history should be elicited from the patient including the presence of dysphagia, regurgitation, chest pain, and heartburn, as well as duration of symptoms and significant weight loss. Symptoms of GERD are often similar to those of a severe dysmotility disorder, most commonly achalasia and less commonly diffuse esophageal spasm. Therefore, when a patient complains of dysphagia, the examiner must know whether it is to solids alone or to both solids and liquids. When liquid dysphagia is a significant part of the history, the patient starts in the upright position, swallowing a small amount of low-density barium. If there is any delay in emptying, or findings suggesting achalasia, such as a dilated esophagus or a bird-beak appearance of the distal esophagus, the patient proceeds to a timed barium swallow.[5] If the examiner starts the study of a patient with unsuspected achalasia with the routine, air-contrast examination, using gas-producing crystals and high-density barium, the subsequent study is largely ruined.

There are multiple phases of a barium esophagram, not all of which need be performed (**Box 1**). It is important to tailor the examination to the patient based on

---

Box 1
Phases of a barium esophagram

- Timed barium swallow (assesses esophageal emptying with the patient in the upright position)
- Upright phase (most often performed using air-contrast techniques)
- Motility phase performed primarily in the right anterior oblique position (performed in the semiprone position)
- Distended or full-column phase performed primarily in the right anterior oblique position (performed in the semiprone position with the patient rapidly drinking)
- Mucosal relief phase (observed at the end of the distended or full-column phase of the examination)
- Reflux assessment (after esophagus has emptied, with the patient in the supine or left posterior oblique position)
- "Solid" food assessment (13 mm barium tablet, marshmallow, or offending food)
- Gastric findings, including emptying (observing the gastric motility fluoroscopically)

condition, signs and symptoms, and ability to ingest various densities of barium, a barium tablet, or various foodstuffs.

THE PREOPERATIVE BARIUM ESOPHAGRAM
Initial Upright Phase

If there is liquid dysphagia, an initial timed barium swallow is performed (**Fig. 1**).[5] With the patient in the upright position, the patient is asked to ingest up to 250 mL of

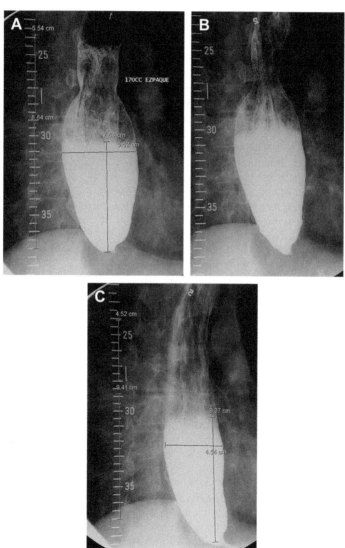

Fig. 1. Timed barium swallow in a patient with type I achalasia. (*A*) One-minute, upright film, with measurements after the patient ingested 170 mL of low-density barium. (*B*) Two-minute, upright film, without measurements. (*C*) Five-minute, upright film, with measurements. There is very little emptying between the 1- and 5 minute films. Unless there has been complete emptying at 2 minutes, the height and width of the barium column is reported at 1 and 5 minutes.

low-density barium. The patient is told that the volume is entirely self-regulated and based on his or her tolerance level. The patient is allowed to ingest the barium over 45 seconds after which an upright spot film is taken, attempting to include the entire barium column on this film. If the column is too high, 2 spot films are take, 1 lower and 1 upper. If barium does not empty, the authors then take 2- and 5-minute films. Unless the barium has emptied in the interval, the 1- and 5-minute films are compared, measuring the height and width of the barium column on both. It is important to keep the image intensifier or tower at the same distance from the patient for all the spot films, so as not to alter the level of magnification. The amount of barium ingested is also recorded. A normal esophagus should empty 250 mL of low-density barium within seconds.

If there is no significant liquid dysphagia, the examination should start with the patient in the upright position, preferably using an air-contrast technique.[2,4] In the authors' practice, the upright position helps in identifying a foreshortened or short esophagus (also known as a fixed, hiatal hernia) (**Fig. 2**).[6-8] Many surgeons, especially thoracic surgeons, consider it important to preoperatively identify a foreshortened esophagus, as this often leads to the addition of a Collis gastroplasty or lengthening procedure, rather than a Nissen fundoplication alone. Their belief is that with a short esophagus the hernia often cannot be completely mobilized and reduced below the diaphragm, especially using abdominal, laparoscopic techniques. If the esophagus is not adequately mobilized and the hernia reduced, the hernia repair is under tension, given the propensity of the foreshortened esophagus to pull back into the mediastinum; this often leads not only to disruption of the hiatus repair and a recurrence of the hernia, but also to a disruption of the fundoplication.[9] It should be noted that not all surgeons believe in the concept of a short esophagus.

In most practices, endoscopy is used to identify reflux esophagitis and Barrett esophagus. Nonetheless, the air-contrast portion of the examination can identify findings of reflux esophagitis and Barrett esophagus, although with much lower sensitivity. The findings of mild reflux esophagitis include a fine nodular or granular mucosal pattern. Changes of moderate to severe reflux esophagitis vary from shallow ulcers and erosions to longitudinal fold thickening and submucosal ridging. Peptic stricture formation is the most significant finding of severe esophagitis.[10] A high esophageal stricture or ulcer and a reticular pattern are strongly associated with Barrett esophagus (**Fig. 3**). Using meticulous technique, the air-contrast portion of the examination can identify patients at low, moderate, or high risk for Barrett esophagitis. In a blinded retrospective study of 200 patients with severe reflux symptoms examined with double-contrast esophagrams and endoscopy, moderate risk was considered present when there was a distal stricture or esophagitis, and high risk if there was a high stricture or ulcer or a reticular pattern.[11] The sensitivity of the esophagram for moderate or severe esophagitis was 71% and for severe esophagitis 85%, with endoscopy detecting only 20 of 46 (43%) of radiographically diagnosed strictures, and with endoscopy failing to identify any stricture not identified on esophagography. Using the esophagram as a method of selecting patients based on moderate or high risk for Barrett esophagus, the overall radiologic sensitivity was 95% (21 of 22) but the specificity was only 65% (116 of 178). The positive predictive value was only 25% (21 of 83) but the negative predictive value was 99% (116 of 117).

If the air-contrast phase cannot be performed, it is still essential to attempt to examine the patient in the upright position with low-density barium to identify a fixed hiatal hernia (ie, foreshortened esophagus).

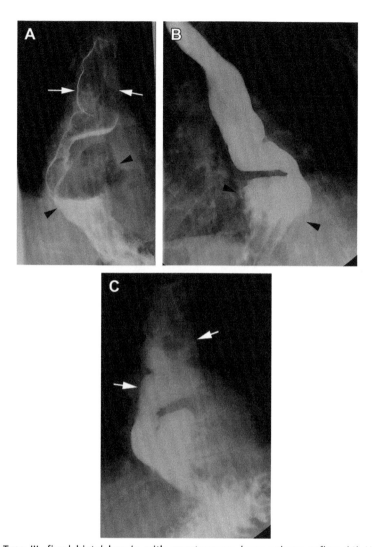

Fig. 2. Type III, fixed hiatal hernia with spontaneous, large-volume reflux. (*A*) Upright, air-contrast spot film showing a large, fixed (nonreducible) hiatal hernia (*black arrowheads*) and a tortuous, patulous esophagus (*white arrows*). (*B*) The large hiatal hernia filled with barium on the full column, semiprone view (*arrowheads*). (*C*) Spontaneous, continuous reflux in the supine position (*white arrows*).

Semiprone or Right Anterior Oblique Phase

The motility portion of the examination is important because it demonstrates the presence and state of peristalsis and bolus transfer, something that only impedance can show.[12] Seminal work by Ott and Richter showed that if 4 of 5 single swallows on a barium esophagram were normal, showing normal bolus transfer in an aboral fashion, then the manometry was normal as well.[13,14] The examiner must focus attention on the inverted V of the tail end of the barium column to properly assess the motility (this corresponds to the upstroke of the pressure wave identified on manometry) (**Fig. 4**). In

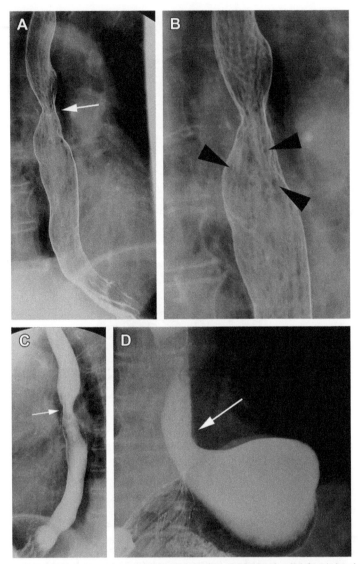

Fig. 3. Barrett stricture in a patient with long-standing GERD and solid-food dysphagia. (*A*) Smooth, tapered narrowing (*white arrow*) at the level of the left pulmonary artery (mid esophagus) on the air-contrast portion of the examination. (*B*) A smaller field-of-view spot film of the air-contrast portion showing nodular folds (*black arrowheads*). (*C*) Persistent, smooth narrowing (*white arrow*) on the semiprone, full-column portion of the examination. (*D*) Spontaneous and continuous reflux (*white arrow*) in the supine portion of the examination. This continuous reflux was present to the level of the cervical esophagus and never cleared.

one retrospective series of 151 patients, the frequency of dysmotility (defined by intermittent weakened or absent peristalsis without or with multiple transient indentations on the barium column as the peristaltic wave traversed the esophagus) was much higher in patients with GERD than in those without.[15]

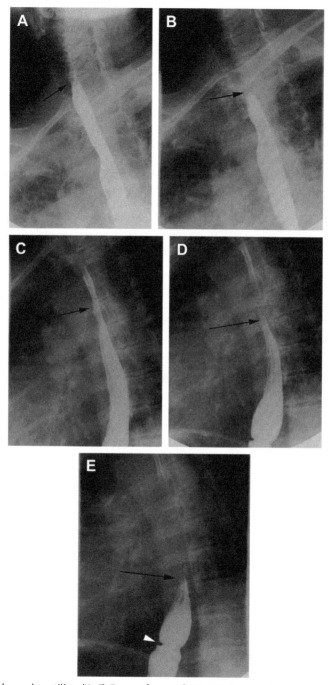

Fig. 4. Esophageal motility. (*A–E*) Freeze frames from a video esophagram demonstrating aboral transmission of the pressure wave distally from the cervical esophagus to the epiphrenic ampulla. The inverted V (*black arrow*) corresponds to the upstroke of the pressure wave. There is some retrograde escape of barium above the inverted V at the juncture of the proximal and middle third of the esophagus (at the juncture of the skeletal and smooth muscle) (*C, D*). This finding is generally not clinically significant unless a large amount escapes above the pressure wave. There is also a distal mucosal ring (*white arrowhead in E*).

With the full implementation of high-resolution manometry and the concurrent use of high-resolution impedance with high-resolution manometry, the impact of the barium assessment of motility has been reduced.[16] The combination of these 2 techniques will show whether low-amplitude peristalsis will have any effect on bolus transit. Regardless, unsuspected and severe motility disorders can be identified during the esophagram, leading to a more detailed analysis with these new techniques. Conversely, if 4 of 5 separate swallows are normal, it is very unlikely that a motility disorder exists.

The full-column, distended, or rapid-drinking phase of the examination identifies overall esophageal distensibility, extrinsic compression or narrowing, strictures, and distal mucosal rings. It may be difficult for patients with long-standing, significant dysphagia to rapidly drink, as they have mentally accommodated over time to not do so. It is important for the examiner to encourage the patient to drink as rapidly as tolerable. During this phase, the authors often slowly pan down the entire course of the esophagus during fluoroscopy, not taking spot films, to identify contour abnormalities and assess the distensibility of the lumen. Special attention should be focused on the distal esophagus, in the region of the epiphrenic ampulla and gastroesophageal junction, a common site of disease. Diffuse, subtle narrowing of the esophagus can result from GERD, but other causes must be considered, especially eosinophilic esophagitis (EOE). EOE is increasingly recognized as a common cause of dysphagia, but unfortunately many of the patients have been misdiagnosed with GERD, as EOE and GERD symptoms overlap.

Directly after the cessation of the rapid drinking is the start of the mucosal relief portion of the examination. This underutilized part of the evaluation is important in several respects. First, the ringed esophagus sometimes present in EOE is often only identified during this phase.[17] Second, thickened esophageal folds from esophagitis are best identified during this phase. If one is unable to adequately coat the esophagus with high-density barium, the only other way to diagnose mild to moderate esophagitis is by identifying fold thickening.

Reflux Identification Phase

The next phase of the examination is to identify gastroesophageal reflux. While the patient remains in the semiprone position, after the mucosal relief stage the esophagus is fluoroscopically assessed for retained barium. If present, the table is raised to the semierect position and the patient is given some water to clear the esophagus of barium. Then, after resuming the horizontal position, the patient is turned to the supine position and the esophagus is examined fluoroscopically. If barium is present in the esophagus, it must have refluxed with motion. If barium is not present the authors proceed with a series of maneuvers starting with a cough or Valsalva maneuver, and then to a water siphon test.

This graded approach in a well-performed investigation increased the sensitivity of identifying reflux when compared with 24-hour pH monitoring studies.[18] When reflux occurs the authors record the cause, if not spontaneous, the height of the reflux (distal, mid, and proximal thoracic and cervical) as well as the length of time the barium remains in the esophagus (<30 or >30 seconds).

This phase of the examination is less important vis-à-vis continuous pH monitoring using a catheter or capsule. However, it is important when there is repeated, continuous, and spontaneous reflux to the cervical esophagus. Trace, intermittent, or low-volume reflux identified on barium studies has little to no clinical significance.

Solid Food Ingestion Phase

The next part of the examination is to assess for the passage of solid food. The authors generally use a 13-mm barium tablet and have the patient ingest the tablet with water. If tablet passage is impaired, the patient ingests low-density barium to identify the precise site and cause, and whether symptoms were elicited (again, before the examination, the patient should be encouraged to voice symptoms if such symptoms occur during the examination). It is common for the tablet to transiently hang up at the level of the transverse aorta and at the level of the gastroesophageal junction. Some institutions administer a standard 30 × 30-mm or a smaller 13 × 12-mm marshmallow (sometimes used in hot chocolate) rather than a 13-mm barium tablet in patients with a distal mucosal ring.[19]

If the patient has consistent dysphagia with a particular food, it is best for the referring physician to have the patient bring that food to the fluoroscopy suite. Ingesting the food, combined with barium paste, can be instructive in 2 ways. First it can show the site and cause of obstruction. More often in the authors' experience, it shows that there is no obstruction. When patients view the examination and sees that there is nothing causing obstruction their anxiety is often relieved, and their often chronic symptoms may resolve.

Feline Esophagus

The feline esophagus is a transient finding on barium esophagrams, most often fleetingly seen during the air-contrast portion of the examination when the esophagus is collapsing. The finding is that of narrowly spaced, transverse folds, giving a crenulated or accordion appearance, a finding caused by contraction of the longitudinal muscles in the esophagus. The cat esophagus has a similar appearance, hence the naming of this finding.

There is controversy as to whether this finding is caused by GERD or is merely associated with GERD. In a recent investigation from the University of Pennsylvania, during a 2-year period 20 of 224 patients examined with a barium esophagram had a feline esophagus,[20] which was detected during barium reflux in 17 of these 20 patients. Gastroesophageal reflux (GER) of barium was present in all 20 patients, of whom 10 had marked GER and 7 moderate GER (marked GER as defined by reflux of barium to or above the thoracic inlet; moderate GER as defined by reflux of barium to the level of the midthoracic esophagus or aortic arch). From this and other investigations, it seems prudent to investigate patients with this finding for the presence of GERD.

Distal Mucosal Ring (Schatzki Ring)

A distal mucosal ring is an idiopathic ridge of tissue composed of mucosa and submucosa located at the gastroesophageal junction (**Fig. 5**). It is often only identified during the semiprone distended phase of the examination,[21] and by definition is associated with a small, often sliding type I hiatal hernia. It was first described by Templeton in 1944, and later reported by Schatzki and Gary and Ingelfinger and Kramer in 1953.[22] Later reports just identify the ring as the Schatzki ring. Because multiple investigators have described the ring, the authors prefer to use the term distal mucosal ring. There is controversy as to the etiology of this redundant tissue, but the finding, like the feline esophagus, is strongly correlated with GERD. Some gastroenterologists recommend that patients with this finding be evaluated for GERD with pH monitoring.[22]

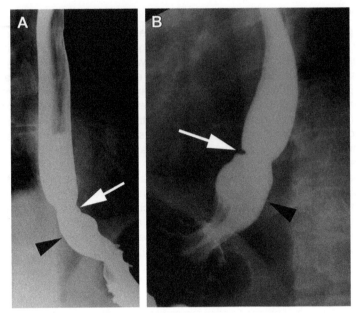

Fig. 5. Small, fixed hiatal hernia with distal mucosal ring in a patient with intermittent solid-food dysphagia. (*A*) Persistent hernia (*black arrowhead*) and narrowing caused at the gastroesophageal junction (*white arrow*) on the upright, air-contrast portion of the examination. (*B*) The same hernia (*black arrowhead*) with the narrowing caused by a mucosal ring (*white arrow*) on the semiprone, full-column portion of the examination.

OUTCOME OF THE PREOPERATIVE EXAMINATION

At the end of the examination, gastroenterologists and esophageal surgeons expect that the radiologist has assessed the level of esophageal emptying in patients with liquid dysphagia (**Box 2**).[3] The presence and type of hiatal hernia should be identified.[23] Type I hernias are sliding-type, small hernias present only in the semiprone position. There is a large degree of subjectivity in the criteria defining a sliding-type or type I hernia using radiography. The radiographic definition is more than a 2 cm separation between the B ring and the diaphragmatic hiatus.[24] Separation less than

---

Box 2
What the gastroenterologist and esophageal surgeon want to know from the preoperative examination

- Assessment of esophageal emptying
- Presence and type of hiatal hernia
- Foreshortening of the esophagus (ie, a hiatal hernia that does not reduce in the upright position)
- Motility: ineffective or absent pump
- Stricture or distal mucosal ring
- Presence, cause, height, and persistence of reflux
- Does the patient have an alternative diagnosis to GERD?

2 cm has been attributed to physiologic herniation. Unfortunately, the B ring is not visible in many patients. In addition, the esophageal gastric junction moves during deglutition because of longitudinal muscle contraction. As a result, the esophagus can shorten approximately 2 cm. Thus, the radiographic identification of a type I hernia is considered unreliable, as is endoscopic identification. Clinically this is not as important as recognizing a fixed hernia.

Type II hernias are rare and are true paraesophageal hernias, with the gastroesophageal junction below the diaphragm and a portion of the fundus herniated through a rent in the diaphragm separate from the hiatus. Type III hernias are the most common paraesophageal hernia and are complex, often large, and associated with a foreshortened esophagus, when a large portion of the fundus is present in the posterior, inferior mediastinum. The herniated stomach may rotate along the vertical (mesoaxial) or horizontal (organoaxial) planes. Type IV hernias are large, complex paraesophageal hernias, which contain not only the stomach but also other organs such as the transverse colon, small bowel, and pancreas. There is a strong association between the size of the hiatal hernia and the presence of reflux.[25]

The presence of a foreshortened esophagus (most often with a fixed or nonreducible hiatal hernia) should be noted. Findings that suggest a short esophagus include a large hernia (>5 cm), a fixed or nonreducible hernia in the upright position, the presence of an esophageal stricture, and nondistensibility of the distal esophagus/epiphrenic ampulla.

A qualitative assessment of the motility should be stated. The most important findings are an ineffective or absent peristalsis. Ineffective motility is suggested by the presence of a primary peristaltic wave but with significant retrograde escape. Retrograde escape is relatively common, and occurs at the juncture of the proximal and middle third of the esophagus, at the level of the transverse aorta. Anatomically this is at the juncture of the skeletal and smooth muscle. Significant retrograde escape is a qualitative judgment, but generally is present when more than half of the barium bolus is not transferred and escapes proximally past this site. When there is no propagation of the primary wave, there is aperistalsis.

The presence and significance of a distal mucosal ring or stricture should also be noted, as well as whether an ingested barium tablet or food has caused obstruction at the level of the narrowing and whether the obstructed tablet or food has caused symptoms. There is a strong relationship between the degree of narrowing of a distal mucosal ring and the presence of symptoms.[19] As the luminal diameter decreases from 20 mm to 9 mm, the likelihood of symptoms from an ingested marshmallow increases. In general, distal mucosal rings larger than 20 mm rarely, if ever, cause symptoms. Rings 13 to 20 mm in diameter variably cause symptoms, with symptoms increasing based on the increasing size of the food bolus. Rings less than 13 mm in diameter invariably cause symptoms regardless of the size of the food bolus.

The presence, cause, height, and persistence (<30 or >30 seconds) of reflux should be noted. Lastly, alternative diagnoses other than GERD should be raised. Two important categories are a severe dysmotility disorder and EOE.

ALTERNATIVE DIAGNOSES TO GERD

The most common severe dysmotility disorders are achalasia and diffuse esophageal spasm. It may be difficult to distinguish the two, but generally achalasia is more easily identified. The barium findings of achalasia include a dilated, aperistaltic esophagus containing foam/saliva, food, and fluid.[26,27] The region of the lower esophageal sphincter can have a bird-beak appearance. Thus, the 2 basic findings of achalasia can be identified: aperistalsis and abnormal relaxation of the lower esophageal sphincter. These findings are typical of the newly classified type I or classic achalasia (based on high-resolution manometry) (impaired relaxation with esophageal dilation and negligible esophageal pressurization).[28] Other findings include vigorous esophageal contractions along with aperistalsis, generally in a normal-caliber esophagus (often type II [panesophageal pressurization] or type III [spastic, contractions of the distal esophageal segment] achalasia). It is often impossible to distinguish achalasia from diffuse esophageal spasm in a patient with these radiographic findings. Furthermore, a normal esophagram may not identify any abnormalities in patients with early achalasia. It is interesting that in a relatively recent investigation from the University of Pennsylvania, 7 of 21 patients with radiographic findings of achalasia on barium esophagrams had complete relaxation of the lower esophageal sphincter (manometry performed was not high-resolution manometry).[27]

EOE is increasingly identified as a common cause of dysphagia, and is more common in men and Caucasian patients. In the authors' experience many patients with EOE have been misidentified as having GERD or a psychogenic cause of their symptoms. Unless the findings on the barium esophagram are identified and confirmed by endoscopy and biopsy, the patients continue to suffer. The findings of EOE on the barium esophagram include: focal esophageal strictures (either single or multiple and relatively equally present in the proximal, mid, and distal esophagus); a ringed esophagus (**Fig. 6**), most commonly identified on collapsed or partially collapsed esophagus; and a small-caliber or diffusely narrowed esophagus.[17,29–32] Any of these findings, especially in the absence of a hiatal hernia, changes of reflux esophagitis, and/or absence of identifiable reflux on the barium examination, should prompt the examiner to consider EOE as the cause.

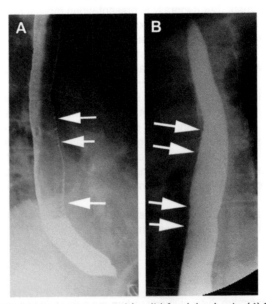

Fig. 6. Ringed esophagus in a young man with solid-food dysphagia. (*A*) Subtle rings (*white arrows*) in the upright, air-contrast portion of the examination. (*B*) These rings (*white arrows*) persist during the semiprone, full-column portion of the examination. Biopsies confirm the presence of eosinophilic esophagitis.

DIAGNOSIS OF ESOPHAGITIS AND BARRETT ESOPHAGUS WITH THE BARIUM ESOPHAGRAM

As previously stated, in some centers an emphasis is placed on the detection of abnormalities strongly associated with Barrett esophagus in an attempt to determine which patients should undergo endoscopy.[11] In a group of 309 patients (including 257 reported cases and unpublished data), Barrett esophagus was associated with the following findings on esophagrams: hiatal hernia (87%), esophageal stricture (72%), thickened folds (65%) on the mucosal relief portion of the examination, gastroesophageal reflux (60%), distal esophageal dilation (44%), esophageal ulcer (40%) and a reticular pattern (23%) (see **Fig. 3**; **Fig. 7**).[33] However, this approach has not been rigorously tested and is based on only on relatively small, retrospective, case series investigations. There has never been a large, prospective study comparing the sensitivity of a well-performed barium esophagram with endoscopy in identifying either moderate to severe esophagitis or Barrett esophagus. Furthermore, the most common abnormality associated with Barrett esophagus is a hiatal hernia, a finding that is very common and thus very nonspecific. It is also unlikely that the esophagram would replace endoscopy in the evaluation of these patients. Thus, in the authors' institution the role of the esophagram in the detection of moderate to severe esophagitis is limited. Nevertheless, if an ulcer, stricture, or thickened folds are identified on the barium study, endoscopy is strongly advised.

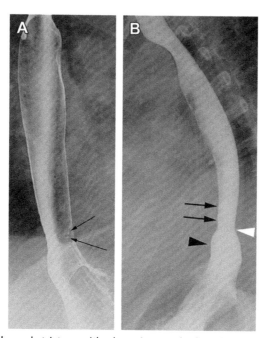

Fig. 7. Distal esophageal stricture with ulcerations and a hiatal hernia. (*A*) Subtle ulcerations (*black arrows*) in the distal esophagus on the upright, air-contrast portion of the examination. (*B*) Diffuse narrowing (nondistensible epiphrenic ampulla) of the distal esophagus (*black arrows*) above the gastroesophageal junction (*white arrowhead*) and a hiatal hernia (*black arrowhead*) on the semiprone, full-column portion of the examination.

THE BARIUM ESOPHAGRAM AFTER ANTIREFLUX PROCEDURES

In the experience of the authors and others, the barium esophagram provides essential information in evaluating symptomatic patients after antireflux procedures.[3,34,35] A careful study best assesses the anatomic problems contributing to these symptoms. At the Cleveland Clinic, all symptomatic post-fundoplication patients have an esophagram as an essential, and usually initial, part of their evaluation.

As with the preoperative examination, eliciting a short history from the patient helps guide the subsequent examination. The authors always ask the patient about the symptoms before the surgery and whether these symptoms were improved or eliminated after the surgery. If the symptoms did not improve after surgery, it is likely that the patient did not have GERD. The patient is also asked about current symptoms, as these often change after the procedure. For instance, a patient may have had severe heartburn before antireflux surgery and developed solid-food dysphagia after the surgery. In such as case the wrap is often too tight.

Initial Upright Phase

If there is any liquid dysphagia, as with the preoperative examination the patient may start by ingesting a small amount of low-density barium to assess for emptying impairment. If there is any delay in emptying, the authors then proceed with a timed barium swallow. Many patients with too tight a wrap have impaired esophageal emptying. This simple test graphically and quantitatively identifies this problem. Furthermore, every year the authors encounter a few patients who have erroneously had a fundoplication in the face of achalasia.

If a timed barium swallow is not performed, the air-contrast phase of the examination begins. An attempt is made to coat the fundoplication so as to identify its length and location vis-à-vis the diaphragm, gastroesophageal junction, and stomach, as well as its integrity. To do so, after the patient ingests the gas-producing crystals and high-density barium and the esophagus is examined upright, the table is rotated to the horizontal position with the patient supine, and the patient is rolled toward the left lateral decubitus position and back again, several times, to fill the posteriorly located fundoplication. Several spot films are taken of the gastroesophageal junction region in multiple planes, even prone. Despite these maneuvers, the best time to examine the wrap is often during the drinking phase of the examination, with the patient in the right anterior oblique position. During this phase, careful attention should be directed to the gastroesophageal junction, diaphragm, and wrap.

Semiprone or Right Anterior Oblique Examination

Motility is then assessed using the standard 5 swallows of low-density barium. In cases where the wrap is too tight, the peristaltic wave may be normal to the level of the epiphrenic ampulla. At this point the epiphrenic ampulla balloons out, and there is retrograde escape of the barium. This process demonstrates that the pressure gradient across the wrap is greater than the pressure of the primary wave.

The distended, full-column or rapid drinking phase of the examination is important in locating and identifying the diaphragm, gastroesophageal junction, gastric fundus, and fundoplication. The authors pay specific attention to this area, attempting to determine: (1) the location of the wrap vis-à-vis the stomach, diaphragm, and esophagus; (2) the integrity and length of the wrap; (3) the lumen the wrap encircles (esophagus, gastroesophageal junction, and/or stomach); and (4) whether there is a recurrent hernia and, if so, its location vis-à-vis the wrap.

Reflux Identification Examination

Next, an attempt is made to identify the presence of reflux using the same maneuvers used in the preoperative patient.

Solid Food Ingestion Examination

The authors then administer the 13-mm barium tablet to determine the tightness of the wrap. The tablet should not obstruct at the level of the fundoplication.

Gastric Motility Assessment

During and at the end of the examination, the motility of the stomach is qualitatively assessed. Unfortunately, the vagus nerve is sometimes damaged during antireflux surgery, which leads to depressed or absent gastric motility, causing bloating, early satiety, and a sense of upper abdominal fullness.

Normal Nissen Fundoplication

A normal Nissen fundoplication should be located below the diaphragm and be no greater than 2 to 3 cm in length (**Fig. 8**).[3,35] The wrap should surround the gastro-esophageal junction and not surround too much of the gastric fundus. There should be no significant narrowing of the lumen at the level of the wrap, and there should not be significant impairment of passage of either a 13-mm tablet or a marshmallow. On single swallows assessing motility, there should be no significant retrograde escape of barium distally, and there should be no significant dilation or ballooning of the esophagus during the rapid drinking phase of the examination. In the upright position, there should be no significant delay in emptying. It may be very difficult to completely opacify a normal fundoplication, as they can be short and small. One will only identify the effect of the wrap on the lumen that is surrounded by the wrap.

Normal Toupet Fundoplication

A Toupet fundoplication is a partial wrap of approximately 270°.[3,35] This uncommon surgery is generally performed in patients with moderate to severe hypomotility. As such, the peristalsis on these patients is often depressed or absent. It may be very difficult to differentiate a Toupet from a Nissen fundoplication on barium examination.

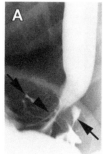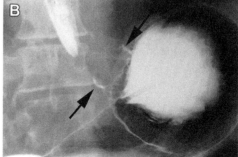

Fig. 8. Normal Nissen fundoplication. (*A*) Small leaves of the fundoplication (*arrows*) encircling the gastroesophageal junction (*arrowhead*) on the semiprone, full-column portion of the examination. (*B*) The leaves of the fundoplication (*arrows*) on a supine view of the fundus.

Collis Gastroplasty–Nissen Fundoplication

A Collis gastroplasty followed by a Nissen fundoplication is performed in patients with foreshortened esophagi.[36,37] In this procedure, lateral stapling of the gastric fundus creates a short neo-esophagus. Thus the distal neo-esophagus is composed of gastric wall and mucosa. A wedge resection of the fundus is often performed to eliminate some of the redundant gastric fundus. The remaining fundus is then used to create the fundoplication. In the authors' experience the fundoplications in patients after a Collis gastroplasty–Nissen procedure are relatively large and "floppy." Knowledge of the presence of a Collis-Nissen procedure is very important to avoid misdiagnosis of a large, long fundoplication or a slipped or malpositioned fundoplication (**Fig. 9**).

After this procedure, in some patients (often with solid-food dysphagia) the 13-mm tablet often obstructs at the level of the gastroplasty or neo-esophagus. In almost all cases, the obstruction is due to a strictured gastroplasty rather than a tight fundoplication (the fundoplications are rarely tight). When the gastroplasty is performed, the blood supply is reduced, often leading to an ischemic stricture.

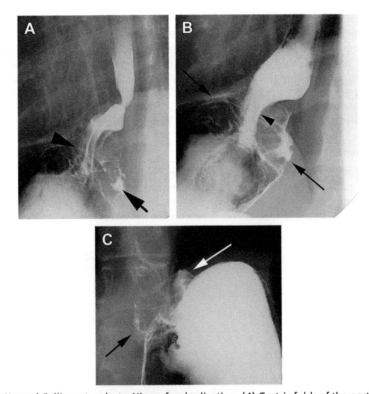

Fig. 9. Normal Collis gastroplasty–Nissen fundoplication. (*A*) Gastric folds of the gastroplasty (neo-esophagus) (*arrowhead*) and one of the leaves of the fundoplication (*arrow*) on the semiprone, full-column portion of the examination. (*B*) A cone-down spot film showing both leaves of the fundoplication (*arrows*) encircling the gastroplasty (*arrowhead*) on the semiprone, full-column portion of the examination. (*C*) The encircling fundoplication (*arrows*) is best shown on a supine view of the fundus.

Abnormal or Failed Fundoplication

As stated previously, it is important for the radiologist to know the preoperative symptoms and whether they resolve after the procedure. It is also important to know whether the postoperative symptoms have recurred or are new. After antireflux surgery, patients may have recurrent heartburn or may have new symptoms of dysphagia, regurgitation, early satiety, or gas-bloat syndrome. It is often easy to predict the radiographic findings based on the patient's postoperative symptoms.

After a Nissen fundoplication patients can present with several findings, a common one being that the fundoplication or wrap is too long and/or too tight and wraps the stomach. This problem often leads to solid-food dysphagia and/or gas bloat (**Fig. 10**). These long, tight wraps surrounding the stomach obstruct the passage of a 13-mm tablet. It is assumed that this failure arises from a poorly formed or malpositioned fundoplication. Another common finding is that the wrap has herniated up into the posterior mediastinum, in a paraesophageal fashion (**Fig. 11**). More often than not, the wrap in these cases is either partially or completely disrupted. In addition, there may be a recurrent hiatal hernia (ie, the gastroesophageal junction is above the diaphragm). The last common finding is that a portion of the stomach is positioned above the wrap, either below or above the diaphragm, with the wrap intact. Some investigators describe this as a slipped Nissen fundoplication. Many surgeons believe that the last 2 findings described are due to failure to recognize a foreshortened esophagus, and/or inadequate mobilization of the esophagus and reduction of the hernia. In some cases the fundoplication may be completely disrupted with recurrence of the hiatal hernia. In unusual cases, incomplete ligation of the short gastric vessels causes rotational tension on the fundoplication, causing a twist at the wrap site.

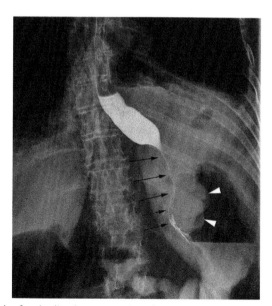

Fig. 10. Long, tight fundoplication, wrapping the stomach in a patient with solid-food dysphagia immediately after surgery. Upright, overhead view of the lower chest and upper abdomen at the end of the examination shows the long fundoplication (*white arrowheads*) wrapping the stomach and causing luminal narrowing (*black arrows*). Note the retained barium in the distal esophagus above the long fundoplication.

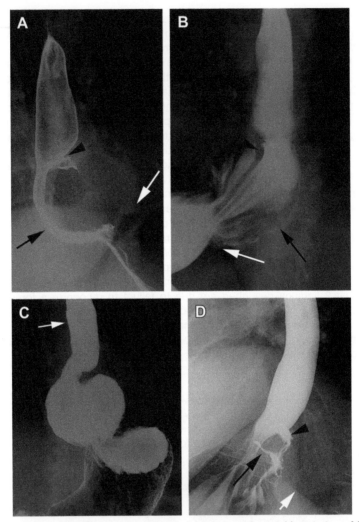

Fig. 11. Status post type III hernia repair with disruption and partial herniation of fundoplication. (*A*) Preoperative fixed, type III hiatal hernia on the upright, air-contrast view (*black arrowhead*, gastroesophageal junction; *black arrow*, hiatal hernia; *white arrow*, diaphragmatic hiatus). (*B*) The same findings on the semiprone, full-column view (*black arrowhead*, gastroesophageal junction; *black arrow*, hiatal hernia; *white arrow*, diaphragmatic hiatus). (*C*) Spontaneous, continuous reflux in the supine position (*white arrow*). (*D, E*) Partially disrupted fundoplication that does not completely encircle the distal esophagus and gastroesophageal junction. A portion of the wrap (*black arrow* in *D* and *E*) is at the level of the diaphragm (*white arrow* in *D*), and a portion of the wrap is above the diaphragm (*black arrowhead* in *D* and *E*). (*F*) A recurrent hiatal hernia with gastric folds above the gastroesophageal junction (*black arrows*). It is likely that either there was too much esophageal foreshortening or there was inadequate esophageal mobilization and hernia reduction, leading to a repair under tension.

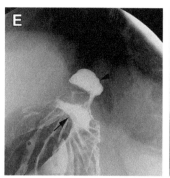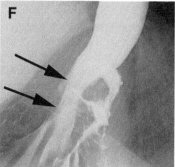

Fig. 11. (*continued*)

OUTCOME OF THE POSTOPERATIVE EXAMINATION

At the end of the examination, gastroenterologists and esophageal surgeons expect that the radiologist has assessed the level of esophageal emptying in patients with liquid dysphagia (**Box 3**),[3] and want a description of: (1) the integrity (intact, partially or completely disrupted) of the wrap; (2) its location vis-à-vis the diaphragm; and (3) which lumen is wrapped. Some investigators have separated the anatomic relationship of the fundoplication vis-à-vis the stomach, esophagus, and diaphragm into various types.[38–40] Because it can be difficult or impossible to easily classify failed fundoplications into neat and tidy types, the authors prefer to describe the individual findings as already described herein. Clinicians also want an assessment of the tightness of the wrap as assessed by the passage of a 13 mm tablet.

In addition to information concerning the fundoplication, the gastroenterologist and, especially, the surgeon expect that a recurrent hiatal hernia is identified. Sometimes the herniated wrap occupies more space in the posterior mediastinum than the recurrent hernia (ie, gastroesophageal junction). An assessment of motility and the presence of recurrent reflux should be reported. Lastly, a qualitative assessment of gastric motility is helpful in identifying the cause of the postoperative bloating or early satiety.

Box 3
What the gastroenterologist and esophageal surgeon want to know from the post-antireflux procedure examination

- Assessment of esophageal emptying
- Fundoplication location vis-à-vis diaphragm
- Fundoplication integrity
- Lumen wrapped by fundoplication
- Fundoplication length
- Fundoplication tightness
- Recurrence of hernia or herniated fundoplication
- Motility
- Gastric emptying

SUMMARY

In their multigroup practice, the authors have found that the barium esophagram forms an integral part of the assessment and management of patients with GERD before and, especially, after antireflux procedures. One could argue that all of the findings revealed by the examination could be identified with endoscopy, a gastric emptying study, and an esophageal motility examination.[41] However, rather than thinking about these examinations as competitors, the authors consider them to be complementary examinations which, when taken as a whole, fully evaluate a patient with suspected GERD as well as symptomatic patients after antireflux procedures.

ACKNOWLEDGMENTS

The authors thank Steven Shay, MD for his helpful and constructive comments and input regarding this article.

REFERENCES

1. Peters JH. Modern imaging for the assessment of gastroesophageal reflux disease begins with the barium esophagram. J Gastrointest Surg 2000;4:346–7.
2. Levine MS, Rubesin SE. Diseases of the esophagus: diagnosis with esophagography. Radiology 2005;237:414–27.
3. Baker ME, Einstein DM, Herts BR, et al. Gastroesophageal reflux disease: integrating the barium esophagram before and after antireflux surgery. Radiology 2007;243:329–39.
4. Levine MS, Rubesin SE, Laufer I. Barium esophagography: a study for all seasons. Clin Gastroenterol Hepatol 2008;6:11–25.
5. deOliveira JM, Birgisson S, Doinoff C, et al. Timed barium swallow: a simple technique for evaluating esophageal emptying in patients with achalasia. AJR Am J Roentgenol 1997;169:473–9.
6. Gastal OL, Hagen JA, Peters JH, et al. Short esophagus. Arch Surg 1999;134:633–8.
7. Mittal SK, Awad ZT, Tasset M, et al. The preoperative predictability of the short esophagus in patients with stricture or paraesophageal hernia. Surg Endosc 2000;14:464–8.
8. Awad ZT, Mittal SK, Roth TA, et al. Esophageal shortening during the era of laparoscopic surgery. World J Surg 2002;25:558–61.
9. Hashemi M, Peters JH, DeMeester TR, et al. Laparoscopic repair of large type III hiatal hernia: objective follow-up reveals high recurrence rate. J Am Coll Surg 2000;190:553–60.
10. Ott DJ. Gastroesophageal reflux disease. Radiol Clin North Am 1994;32:1147–66.
11. Gilchrist AM, Levine MS, Carr RF, et al. Barrett's esophagus: diagnosis by double-contrast esophagography. AJR Am J Roentgenol 1988;150:97–102.
12. Cho YK, Choi MG, Baik CN, et al. Comparison of bolus transit patterns identified by esophageal impedance to barium esophagram in patients with dysphagia. Dis Esophagus 2012;25:17–25.
13. Ott DJ, Chen YM, Hewson EG, et al. Esophageal motility: assessment with synchronous video tape fluoroscopy and manometry. Radiology 1989;173:419–22.
14. Hewson EG, Ott DJ, Dalton CB, et al. Manometry and radiology. Complementary studies in the assessment of esophageal motility disorders. Gastroenterology 1990;98:626–32.
15. Campbell C, Levine MS, Rubesin SE, et al. Association between esophageal dysmotility and gastroesophageal reflux on barium studies. Eur J Radiol 2006;59:88–92.

16. Bulsiewicz WJ, Kahrilas PJ, Kwiatek MA, et al. Esophageal pressure topography criteria indicative of incomplete bolus clearance: a study using high resolution impedance manometry. Am J Gastroenterol 2009;104:2721–8.
17. Zimmerman SL, Levine MS, Rubesin SE, et al. Idiopathic eosinophilic esophagitis in adults: the ringed esophagus. Radiology 2005;236:159–65.
18. Thompson JK, Koehler RE, Richter JE. Detection of gastroesophageal reflux: value of barium studies compared with 24-hr pH monitoring. AJR Am J Roentgenol 1994;162:621–6.
19. Smith DF, Ott DJ, Gelfand DW, et al. Lower esophageal mucosal ring: correlation of referred symptoms with radiographic findings using a marshmallow bolus. AJR Am J Roentgenol 1998;171:1361–5.
20. Samadi F, Levine MS, Rubesin SE, et al. Feline esophagus and gastroesophageal reflux. AJR Am J Roentgenol 2010;194:972–6.
21. Ott DJ, Chen YM, Wu WC, et al. Radiographic and endoscopic sensitivity in detecting lower esophageal mucosal ring. AJR Am J Roentgenol 1986;147:261–5.
22. Jalil S, Castell DO. Schatzki's ring; a benign cause of dysphagia in adults. J Clin Gastroenterol 2002;35:295–8.
23. Kahrilas PJ, Kim HC, Pandolfino JE. Approaches to the diagnosis and grading of hiatal hernia. Best Pract Res Clin Gastroenterol 2008;22:601–16.
24. Ott DJ, Gelfand DW, Chen YM, et al. Predictive relationship of hiatal hernia to reflux esophagitis. Gastrointest Radiol 1985;10:317–20.
25. Ott DJ, Glauser SJ, Ledbetter MS, et al. Association of hiatal hernia and gastroesophageal reflux: correlation between presence and size of hiatal hernia and 24-hour pH monitoring of the esophagus. AJR Am J Roentgenol 1995;165:557–9.
26. Blam ME, Delfyett W, Levine MS, et al. Achalasia: a disease of varied and subtle symptoms that do not correlate with radiographic findings. Am J Gastroenterol 2002;97:1916–23.
27. Amaravadi R, Levine MS, Rubesin SE, et al. Achalasia with complete relaxation of lower esophageal sphincter: radiographic-manometric correlation. Radiology 2005;235:886–91.
28. Richter JE. Achalasia—an update. J Neurogastroenterol Motil 2010;16:232–42.
29. Picus D, Frank PH. Eosinophilic esophagitis. AJR Am J Roentgenol 1981;136:1001–3.
30. Vitellas KM, Bennett WF, Bova JG, et al. Idiopathic eosinophilic esophagitis. Radiology 1993;186:789–93.
31. Levine MS, Saul SH. Idiopathic eosinophilic esophagitis: how common is it? Radiology 1993;186:631–2.
32. White SB, Levine MS, Rubesin SE, et al. The small-caliber esophagus: radiographic sign of idiopathic eosinophilic esophagitis. Radiology 2010;256:127–34.
33. Chen MY, Frederick MG. Barrett esophagus and adenocarcinoma. Radiol Clin North Am 1994;32:1167–81.
34. LeBlanc-Louvry I, Koning E, Zalar A, et al. Severe dysphagia after laparoscopic fundoplication: usefulness of barium meal examination to identify causes other than tight fundoplication – a prospective study. Surgery 2000;128:392–8.
35. Canon CL, Morgan DE, Einstein DM, et al. Surgical approach to gastroesophageal reflux disease: what the radiologist needs to know. Radiographics 2005;25:1485–99.
36. Stirling MC, Orringer MB. Continued assessment of the combined Collis-Nissen operation. Ann Thorac Surg 1989;47:224–30.

37. Pierre AF, Luketich JD, Fernando HC, et al. Results of laparoscopic repair of giant paraesophageal hernias: 200 consecutive patients. Ann Thorac Surg 2002;74: 1909–16.
38. Hainaux B, Sattari A, Coppens E, et al. Intrathoracic migration of the wrap after laparoscopic Nissen fundoplication: radiologic evaluation. AJR Am J Roentgenol 2002;178:859–62.
39. Hatch KF, Daily MF, Christensen BJ, et al. Failed fundoplications. Am J Surg 2004; 188:786–91.
40. Richter JE. Gastroesophageal reflux disease treatment: side effects and complications of fundoplication. Clin Gastroenterol Hepatol 2013;11:465–71.
41. Linke GR, Borovicka J, Schneider P, et al. Is a barium swallow complementary to endoscopy essential in the preoperative assessment of laparoscopic antireflux and hiatal hernia surgery? Surg Endosc 2008;22:96–100.

Esophageal Manometry in Gastroesophageal Reflux Disease

Michael Mello, MD, C. Prakash Gyawali, MD*

KEYWORDS

- High-resolution manometry • Esophageal hypomotility
- Hypotensive lower esophageal sphincter • Preoperative testing
- Multiple rapid swallows

KEY POINTS

- High-resolution manometry (HRM) is an effective tool to study pathophysiologic motor events in gastroesophageal reflux disease (GERD).
- HRM has clinical utility in excluding esophageal outflow obstruction mimicking GERD.
- Preoperative esophageal HRM can alter surgical decisions and is of clinical value before antireflux surgery.
- Provocative testing during HRM may assess esophageal smooth muscle peristaltic reserve.

INTRODUCTION

High-resolution manometry (HRM) marks a major advance in the clinical evaluation of esophageal motor disorders. HRM topographic contour plots, known as Clouse plots, are more intuitive than conventional manometry waveform recordings, allowing for pattern recognition and utilization of software tools for interrogation, thereby reducing interobserver variance in interpretation.[1,2] This article discusses the use of HRM in evaluating patients with GERD symptoms in terms of both manometric correlates of GERD and motor findings useful in preoperative assessment for antireflux surgery.

ADVANCES IN ESOPHAGEAL MANOMETRY

Manometry systems are designed to measure the timing and amplitude of pressure events in the esophagus and its sphincters via a linear array of pressure sensors on a catheter. Assimilation, integration, and display systems convert these pressure recordings into electrical signals that can be displayed as pressure waveforms or topographic pressure plots. The roots of HRM began in the mid-1970s when the first

Division of Gastroenterology, Washington University School of Medicine, Campus Box 8124, 660 South Euclid Avenue, St Louis, MO 63110, USA
* Corresponding author.
E-mail address: cprakash@wustl.edu

Gastroenterol Clin N Am 43 (2014) 69–87
http://dx.doi.org/10.1016/j.gtc.2013.11.005
0889-8553/14/$ – see front matter © 2014 Elsevier Inc. All rights reserved.

high-fidelity manometry system was developed by Jerry Dodds and Ron Arndorfer.[3] This initial system was composed of water-perfused catheters, a pneumohydraulic pump, pressure transducers, and a strip-chart recorder with side holes spaced at 3- to 5-cm intervals. The apparatus was later modified by replacement of the strip-chart recordings with digital-analog converters and a video display on computer screens. Manometry subsequently evolved to the use of solid-state catheters, allowing for circumferential pressure averaging and finer evaluation of the pharynx and upper esophageal sphincter (UES) because of a faster frequency response that was better at sensing striated muscle contraction.[4] Critical to the evaluation of the esophagogastric junction (EGJ), a 6-cm perfused sensor called the Dent sleeve was developed in 1976, which increased the ability of the manometry catheter to remain within the LES during esophageal movement,[5] thereby increasing accuracy in LES assessment.

A major step forward occurred in the 1990s when Ray E. Clouse envisioned and developed HRM.[6] This advance involved a vast increase in sensors on the esophageal manometry catheter, generating pressure data that could be displayed as a spatiotemporal plot using color contours to designate pressures (**Fig. 1**). Modern HRM systems use circumferential solid-state sensors 1 cm apart, as well as custom assimilation and display software that allows intuitive interpretation using software tools. Because pressure phenomena from the entire esophagus can be visualized at once, sphincters can be easily identified, thus rendering the stationary pull-through maneuver obsolete.[6] Identification of LES relaxation errors improved, and achalasia is now diagnosed with better accuracy.[4] The technique also provided new insights into gastroesophageal reflux disease (GERD) by refining manometric correlates for the condition, both static (LES basal pressures, hiatus hernia) and dynamic (esophageal peristaltic performance), thereby serving as a useful tool in preoperative evaluation before antireflux surgery.[7] In recent years, the Chicago Classification created new standards by which researchers and clinicians analyze Clouse plots to better describe esophageal motor phenomena.[8] However, the Chicago Classification remains fluid and evolving, and new parameters continue to be designed that better evaluate pressure phenomena in the context of GERD.

PATHOPHYSIOLOGIC CORRELATES OF GERD ON HRM

By the Montreal definition, GERD develops when the reflux of stomach contents causes troublesome symptoms and/or complications.[9] The disease is common worldwide and reduces the quality of life.[10] Proton-pump inhibitors (PPIs) are the mainstay of GERD management, working by binding to the H^+,K^+-ATPase enzyme in the gastric parietal cell to decrease the production of gastric acid. Although this medication class is excellent at suppressing acid production, 30% to 40% of GERD patients continue to have symptoms because the medication does not reverse the pathophysiology of GERD,[11,12] since transient lower esophageal sphincter relaxations (TLESRs), thought to be the critical motor event leading to GERD, are not affected by PPIs. Though physiologically useful in allowing uncomfortable gas release from the stomach, TLESRs are pathologic when gastric contents escape into the lower esophagus, leading to symptoms and mucosal injury.

Transient Lower Esophageal Sphincter Relaxations

Early manometric studies demonstrated a higher proportion of TLESRs accompanied by acid reflux in GERD patients in comparison with controls. Holloway and colleagues[13,14] defined objective conventional manometric criteria for detecting TLESRs,

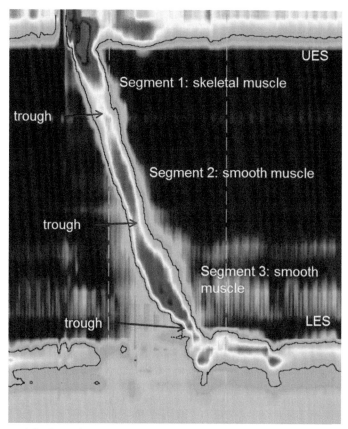

Fig. 1. Normal high-resolution manometry swallow sequence. The topographic plot is anchored by 2 bands of pressure, the upper esophageal sphincter (UES) and the lower esophageal sphincter (LES). Sphincter relaxation with swallows is depicted by dissipation of bright colors to the background blue, which represents low pressures. The peristaltic sequence consists of a chain of contracting segments, the skeletal muscle segment (segment 1), and 2 smooth muscle segments (segments 2 and 3).

which included the following: absence of swallow, rate of relaxation, nadir LES pressure, duration of LES relaxation, crural diaphragm inhibition, and prominent LES after-contraction. These criteria, though initially developed for conventional manometry, have also been used to determine the ability of HRM to detect TLESRs. The manometric signature of a reflux event is the common cavity, defined as a simultaneous intraesophageal pressure increase to gastric pressure levels.[15] pH and pH-impedance studies segregate common cavity events occurring with and without reflux of gastric content.[16] These comparative studies show that HRM is at least equal to, if not superior to conventional manometry in evaluating TLESRs, particularly those accompanied by true reflux.[16–19] Sensitivity for detecting TLESRs associated with reflux is reported to be 96% for HRM and 86% for conventional manometry.[18] The advantage of HRM consists of higher interobserver concordance than conventional manometry (72% vs 25%).[19] Further, HRM also demonstrates that postprandial TLESRs are associated with acid reflux more often than those during fasting, particularly in GERD patients, with increased intragastric pressures during and in the 3 minutes before a TLESR.[16]

Therefore, HRM can replace conventional manometry in the evaluation of TLESRs. However, in clinical evaluation of GERD patients the frequency of TLESRs during a time-limited recording may have less predictive value for patient management than the assessment of the consequence of TLESRs; that is, abnormal pH or reflux parameters on ambulatory pH or pH-impedance monitoring. Therefore, enumeration and evaluation of TLESRs is mostly used in the research setting. Newer motility systems show promise in long-term ambulatory recordings over several hours or even a full day, which may provide overall better understanding of reflux mechanisms.[20]

Barrier Function of the Esophagogastric Junction

EGJ opening with reflux events

HRM has provided a more complete understanding of physiologic EGJ opening and barrier function critical for reflux prevention.[21] Using a combination of HRM, pH probe, endoscopic clips placed at the squamocolumnar junction and 10 cm proximal to the junction, and fluoroscopic examination in the postprandial state, Pandolfino and colleagues[21] demonstrated profound diaphragmatic crural inhibition during TLESRs with reflux, 60% of which occurred during inspiration rather than expiration. Longitudinal muscle contraction in the distal esophagus resulted in esophageal shortening visualized on both manometry and fluoroscopy, and the squamocolumnar junction moved proximal to the crural diaphragm in most instances. LES relaxation was halted by secondary peristalsis (56%), isolated contractions at the distal esophagus (17%), or primary peristalsis (27%). Few reflux episodes fulfilling manometric criteria were confirmed by the pH electrode placed 5 cm above the EGJ, supporting previous observations of the low yield of pH studies in detecting short-segment distal esophageal reflux events.[21,22] Moreover, crural diaphragm function was reduced in patients with objective evidence of GERD when compared with controls and patients without objective evidence of reflux, and that reduced inspiratory EGJ pressure augmentation was an independent predictor of GERD.[14] When the threshold value for inspiratory augmentation was 10 mm Hg, the sensitivity of predicting EGD or pH-positive GERD was 57% while specificity was 79%.[23,24]

In these studies, fluoroscopy is used to localize the squamocolumnar junction following endoscopic clip placement. A new technique using an endoscopically placed magnetic clip at the squamocolumnar junction and a nasally placed probe alongside the HRM catheter continuously follows the location of the squamocolumnar junction during physiologic and pathologic LES events.[25] This technique works through the Hall effect, using voltage changes on a semiconductor around the magnetic field generated by the magnetized clip to generate a digital signal that can be superimposed on the HRM Clouse plot.[25] These and other studies show that both LES (and consequently EGJ) basal pressure and the crural diaphragm contribute to the EGJ barrier function. With TLESRs, in addition to LES opening, distal esophageal shortening from longitudinal muscle contraction and a gastroesophageal pressure gradient are essential for reflux to occur. HRM provides an intuitive image-based paradigm in the evaluation of these pathophysiologic correlates of GERD. It complements other contemporary techniques, including fluoroscopy, pH and pH-impedance monitoring, and high-frequency ultrasonography in the study of TLESRs and the LES-diaphragmatic relationship as a barrier function.[26]

Pressure inversion point and hiatus hernia

A disrupted barrier can consist of low LES pressures as well as a separation between LES and the crural diaphragm. Both of these entities are well recognized on clinical HRM studies.[7,27,28] The crural diaphragm is visually identified by the pressure signature of inspiratory crural contraction. The plane of pressure inversion between the intrathoracic and intra-abdominal cavities is identified by following color contours generated by intraluminal pressures between swallows in the esophageal and gastric lumens during respiration. Finally, a pressure inversion point (PIP) tool is used to interrogate the respiratory pressure inversion point, which can be moved across the LES high-pressure zone and EGJ to identify the precise plane where pressure inverses. Based on the degree of separation between the LES and the diaphragmatic crura as well as the location of the PIP, Pandolfino and colleagues[23] characterize the EGJ findings with respiration into 4 categories (**Fig. 2**). It is currently unclear as to whether these designations affect management decisions in GERD.

HRM allows better understanding of the dynamic nature of the relationship between the LES and the diaphragmatic crura, with spontaneous formation and reduction of hiatal hernias as measured by the separation between the LES diaphragmatic crura.[24] Furthermore, HRM may be more accurate than endoscopy in recording the presence of a hiatus hernia. A study assessing endoscopic and HRM diagnosis of axial hiatus hernias greater than 2 cm in size in comparison with diagnosis at surgery documents that despite comparable sensitivity, HRM has higher specificity than endoscopy, with fewer false positives (5% vs 32%; $P = .01$). This study also describes that HRM has good value in both ruling in and ruling out the presence of an axial hiatus hernia.[29]

In the presence of a large hiatus hernia, the tip of the manometry catheter may coil up within the hiatus hernia and not traverse the diaphragmatic crura. Despite this situation occurring about half the time in hiatus hernias longer than 5 cm,[30,31] interrogation of the esophageal body motor pattern and the LES remains possible, and this is not considered a critical imperfection of the study.[32] The distribution of esophageal body motor disorders in this setting is no different from that observed in patients without a hiatus hernia.[30] However, an important point is to clarify that the pressure within the hiatus hernia is not elevated above the gastric baseline. Because the integrated relaxation pressure (IRP) is measured above the gastric baseline, elevated intrahernia pressures with pressure trapping within hiatus hernia will falsely lower the IRP if the gastric baseline is measured within the hiatus hernia.[31,32] In these instances, placement of the catheter under endoscopic guidance may be warranted.

LES hypotension

A low LES end expiratory pressure is seen more often in GERD patients with regurgitation, those with medically refractory heartburn, and those being evaluated for antireflux surgery (**Fig. 3**).[7,33] The end-expiratory pressure is chosen as the metric for assessing resting LES pressure, recorded when diaphragmatic crura are relaxed and not contributing to the recorded pressure. A period of quiet rest and normal respiration is used for recording basal sphincter parameters at the beginning of the HRM study, making sure no TLESRs, dry swallows, or other artifacts occur within 30 seconds of the landmark recording period.[32] In a large cohort of subjects referred for preoperative HRM before antireflux surgery, Chan and colleagues[7] reported that the proportion of patients with end-expiratory LES pressure of 5 mm Hg or less was 34.1% in the setting of an abnormal ambulatory pH study, and 13.5% when the pH study was normal. The overall likelihood of LES hypotension in the surgical GERD population was 47.1%.

Esophageal Clearance

Esophageal hypomotility is a motor phenomenon evident on esophageal manometry in the setting of GERD, which, when present, may affect clearance of the refluxate and prolong acid contact with esophageal mucosa. Several terms have been used to

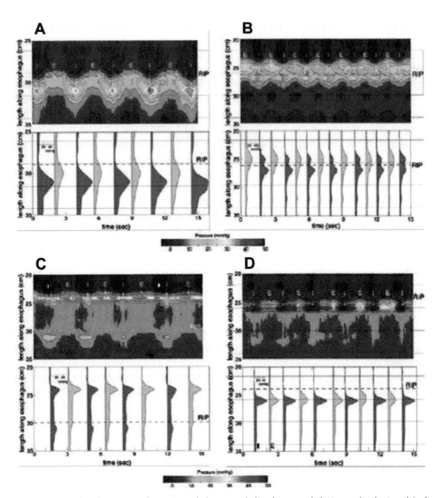

Fig. 2. Relationship between the LES and the crural diaphragm. (*A*) Normal relationship between LES and crural diaphragmatic contractions, with both entities superimposed (type I). The dashed line representing the respiratory pressure inversion point (RIP) lies at the proximal extent of the LES high-pressure zone. (*B*) Minimal separation between the LES and the crural diaphragm, with the RIP at the proximal extent of the crural diaphragm (type II). (*C*) Separation of more than 2 cm between LES and crural diaphragm, with the RIP just proximal to the crural diaphragm (type IIIa). (*D*) Similar separation, but with the RIP just proximal to the LES (type IIIb). Bottom plots under each high-resolution manometry image demonstrate corresponding spatial variation plots (light gray = expiration, dark gray = inspiration) at the planes marked E and I for expiration and inspiration, respectively. (*From* Pandolfino JE, Kim H, Ghosh SK, et al. High-resolution manometry of the EGJ: an analysis of crural diaphragm function in GERD. Am J Gastroenterol 2007;102:1059; with permission.)

describe this phenomenon, including ineffective esophageal motility (IEM) with conventional manometry, and descriptive breaks in the peristaltic contour with HRM.[8,34] Mechanistically, GERD may lead to hypomotility through direct gastric acid exposure, causing esophageal injury and hypomotility. In turn, hypomotility can exacerbate GERD and predispose to erosive disease through decreased clearance of refluxed acidic contents from the distal esophagus. Peristalsis of weak contraction amplitude,

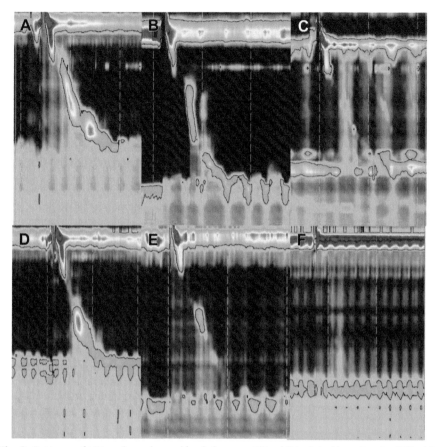

Fig. 3. Patterns of LES and esophageal body hypomotility. (*A*) Isolated hypotensive LES with intact esophageal body peristalsis. (*B*) Small breaks in the peristaltic contour. (*C*) Large break in the peristaltic contour. (*D*) Transition zone defect between skeletal and smooth muscle contraction segments. (*E*) Transition zone defect and a large break in the peristaltic contour. (*F*) Aperistalsis. *B*, *C*, *D*, and *E* represent fragmentation of the peristaltic sequence.

typically less than 30 mm Hg in the distal esophagus, is designated IEM in the esophageal body with conventional manometry.[34] In addition, proportions of failed sequences are reported in this context (see **Fig. 3**).

HRM provides a more detailed topographic map of smooth muscle contraction. Two smooth muscle contraction segments are identified: the proximal (segment 2) with predominantly cholinergic influences, and the distal (segment 3) with predominantly inhibitory influences.[1,4] Several correlates of esophageal hypomotility are identifiable on an HRM study. The first of these are transition-zone defects (see **Fig. 3**). Though also present in normal subjects, transition-zone defects (intersegmental troughs) between striated and smooth muscle contraction segments are identified in hypomotility states including GERD.[35,36] These defects are abnormal or visible breaks in the peristalsis contour between these contraction segments. As much as 93% of subjects evaluated had at least 1 identifiable transition-zone defect, so the mere presence of these defects does not imply hypomotility. However, extended transition-zone defects larger than 3 cm were reported more often in GERD patients

(45%) than in normal controls and patients without GERD (27%), indicating that extended defects may represent hypomotility. This finding may result from poor formation of adjacent contraction segments, particularly the second segment.[36] Timing of initiation of the second segment measured from initiation of the first segment (termed proximal latency) was delayed longer than 4 seconds in 36% of GERD patients, compared with 20% of healthy controls and 19% of patients without GERD.[36] This result supports the fact that extended transition-zone defects may be associated with delayed onset of smooth muscle contraction, and may represent a hypomotility feature seen more often in the setting of GERD.[36]

Another HRM characteristic of esophageal hypomotility is fragmentation of the smooth muscle contraction pattern, resulting in prominent troughs (breaks) between smooth muscle contraction segments (see **Fig. 3**; **Table 1**). Sometimes one of the contraction segments, particularly the second segment, may fail to form, resulting in large breaks in the peristaltic contour.[37] When both segments fail to form, the sequence is designated as failed. Within the Chicago Classification algorithm, a threshold of 20 mm Hg is used to designate failure of peristalsis, because HRM studies combined with stationary impedance demonstrated that bolus transit may be facilitated by sequences that can generate 20 mm Hg of pressure in the esophageal body.[38] Breaks in the peristaltic contour of less than 2 cm at 20 mm Hg and less than 3 cm at 30 mm Hg were found not to affect esophageal bolus clearance.[38] Although failure of contraction has been characterized with conventional manometry in GERD, fragmentation of the peristaltic contour has only been recognized with the use of HRM.[37]

Comparison of the frequency of fragmentation of smooth muscle contraction segments demonstrated that patients with documented GERD, particularly those with Barrett esophagus, were more likely to demonstrate fragmented sequences when compared with controls and those without GERD, similar to the gradient in failed sequences.[37] Patients with GERD also demonstrated lower peak and averaged

Table 1
HRM parameters and metrics useful in the evaluation of the GERD patient

Category	Parameter or Metric
Clinical	
Anatomic	Esophageal length
	Size of hiatus hernia
	LES length
	Length of intra-abdominal LES
LES	End-expiratory LES pressure
	Postswallow residual pressure (IRP)
Esophageal body	Contraction amplitudes
	Distal contractile integral (DCI)
	Transition zone defect, breaks, fragmentation
	Degree of hypomotility[a]
	Response to multiple rapid swallows (MRS)
Research	
LES	Transient lower esophageal sphincter relaxations (TLESRs)
	LES pressure integral, EGJ contractile integral
	3-Dimensional structure of the LES
Esophageal body	Response to provocative maneuvers

[a] See **Table 2**.

contraction amplitudes in the esophageal body in comparison with controls and those without GERD. Whereas 8% of controls demonstrated fragmented sequences, 18% of GERD patients and 25% of those with Barrett esophagus demonstrated this finding. A combination of 30% failed or fragmented sequences could segregate GERD patients from controls (34% GERD patients, 8.4% controls; $P = .04$); 70% of those with Barrett esophagus met this threshold. When fragmented, the second esophageal segment was more likely than the third segment to be compromised (diminished or absent in 82%). These findings support the identification of fragmented and failed sequences as markers of esophageal hypomotility (**Fig. 4**).[37]

Esophageal Length and Other Anatomic Considerations

HRM also allows quick assessment of esophageal length from UES to LES (see **Table 1**).[6] There is proximal migration of the LES with GERD, typically concurrent with formation and enlargement of hiatus hernia. Esophageal length is a metric that is useful for the foregut surgeon in planning antireflux surgery, as a shortened esophagus may require an esophageal lengthening procedure to ensure intra-abdominal location of the LES following antireflux surgery. Although this metric can be obtained from the barium swallow examination, HRM complements this assessment.

The length of the LES and, particularly, the length of the intra-abdominal segment of the LES, can be measured (see **Table 1**).[27] However, there is considerable variability in these metrics, partly depending on the presence or absence of the hiatus hernia. Because of the averaging of pressures from sensors within an asymmetric sphincter, measurement of sphincter length does not demonstrate particular gains with HRM over conventional manometry,[39] despite the fact that the sphincter can be better localized with HRM. In particular, the length of the intra-abdominal segment is overestimated, and sphincter length can vary throughout the study.[39] The use of 3-dimensional manometry with higher density of pressure sensors and sector averaging of pressures (in contrast to circumferential averaging with HRM) can provide a more accurate spatiotemporal map of the LES high-pressure zone,[40] and potentially could develop into a useful research tool (see **Table 1**). However, this technique is not widely available, and to date has not demonstrated advantages over HRM that would have an impact on management decisions.

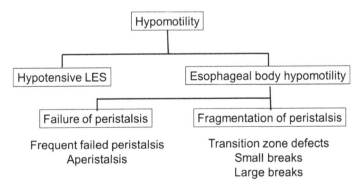

Fig. 4. Proposed classification of hypomotility. Hypomotility can be isolated to the esophageal body or lower esophageal sphincter (LES), or the two can coexist. Esophageal body hypomotility can consist of varying degrees of failure of peristalsis, or fragmentation of the peristaltic sequence, with transition zone defects, and small and large breaks in the peristaltic contour.

HRM SOFTWARE TOOLS AND METRICS

The most impactful HRM software tool is the electronic sleeve used in the assessment of LES postswallow residual pressures.[1,4] The area interrogated by this tool can be adjusted by the user to include the entire LES high-pressure zone, including the crural diaphragm when the 2 are in close proximity. IRP is the metric demonstrated to have the highest sensitivity in segregating normal from abnormal bolus flow across the LES-EGJ, using a threshold of 15 mm Hg.[41] The IRP reports the nadir LES pressure during LES relaxation within the period assessed by the electronic sleeve, averaged over a period of 4 continuous or discontinuous seconds. Assessment of the IRP and determination of EGJ relaxation is the first step in the analysis of HRM studies, and is the starting point for the Chicago Classification algorithm.[4,8] In the context of GERD, the IRP establishes that there is no esophageal outflow obstruction mimicking GERD symptoms, an essential step in excluding achalasia spectrum disorders and esophageal outflow obstruction before antireflux surgery.[7]

HRM software tools have been used in the assessment of vigor of contraction in the smooth muscle esophagus (see **Table 1**). The distal contractile integral (DCI) describes the totality of esophageal smooth muscle contraction in terms of length of the contracting segment, amplitude of contraction, and duration of contraction, measured as mm Hg.cm.s.[42] The upper threshold of normal is 5000 mm Hg.cm.s, established as a mean over 10 water swallows. However, the lower threshold has not been investigated in describing hypomotility. Using statistical modeling to evaluate DCI thresholds, an averaged DCI threshold of 450 mm Hg.cm.s had 78% positive agreement and 83% negative agreement with ineffective swallows, fulfilling a designation of IEM. This study concluded that 5 sequences with breaks or failure of peristalsis with an averaged DCI of less than 450 mm Hg.cm.s could be used to define IEM.[43] This metric shows promise in the designation of severe hypomotility, and may complement other existing metrics (**Table 2**), but there is a lack of outcome data to determine whether this actually influences management decisions.

Use of the DCI metric assessed separately for each of the 2 smooth muscle segments has been found to be helpful in the differential comparison of these segments. Staiano and Clouse[44] reported augmentation of the second segment with the use of cisapride, a procholinergic agent. The authors' group also demonstrated that the 2 smooth muscle contraction segments have equal vigor of contraction in GERD manifesting as chest pain, with a ratio similar to that of normal controls.[45] However, in patients with acid sensitivity (as identified by symptom reflux correlation in the setting of

Table 2
Proposed description of esophageal smooth muscle peristaltic function

	Esophageal Body[a]	Failed Sequences (%)	Implications for Antireflux Surgery
Normal peristalsis	Adequate	≤ 30	None
Mild hypomotility	Adequate	30–50	Probably none[b]
Moderate hypomotility	Adequate	50–70	Probably none[b]
Moderate hypomotility	Inadequate	50–70	Avoid 360° fundoplication
Severe hypomotility	Any	≥ 80	Avoid 360° fundoplication

[a] Adequate: >30 mm Hg averaged amplitudes in the smooth muscle esophagus, or averaged distal contractile integral >450 mm Hg.cm.s for transmitted sequences.
[b] Presence of preoperative dysphagia and lack of contraction response to provocative measures may modify this recommendation.

normal esophageal acid exposure off PPI), the third segment had statistically higher vigor of contraction compared with the second segment. A distal shift in contraction vigor therefore may be a marker for acid sensitivity. Alternatively, the presence of vigorous contraction in the distal esophagus may ensure efficient clearance of refluxate, such that acid exposure times are in the normal range despite symptom reflux association.[45]

A DCI-like metric is now garnering interest in evaluating the resting LES-EGJ pressure. Using the DCI algorithm of contraction vigor, the LES is interrogated during a 10-second basal period, termed the LES pressure integral.[46] The original report suggested that this metric could segregate patients with distal esophageal acid exposure from those without, but the metric was not standardized to gastric pressure or to the respiratory cycle. A further advancement of this technique is to standardize the time duration of the metric to the respiratory cycle, measuring this for exactly 3 cycles, and to the gastric baseline. This metric, termed the EGJ contractile integral, could segregate PPI nonresponders with a regurgitation-predominant reflux phenotype from normal controls and other PPI nonresponder phenotypes. This notion suggests that the EGJ contractile integral segregates a disrupted EGJ barrier from a normotensive LES.[47] However, it is unclear as to how this metric would perform when the LES is separated from the diaphragmatic crura, and whether it would be useful in predicting outcome after therapy for GERD, particularly antireflux surgery, or in assessing the EGJ after fundoplication, as no studies currently exist.

CLINICAL APPLICATION OF HRM METRICS

Although manometry cannot be used to diagnose GERD, HRM findings may be useful in identifying certain pathophysiologic correlates relevant to patient management. As manometry is used for identifying the proximal margin of the LES for placement of pH and pH-impedance catheters, HRM studies are easily available in GERD patients undergoing pH monitoring.[48] Comparative interpretation can be performed in this setting, providing useful insights into esophageal motor patterns with and without abnormal acid exposure. For instance, proportions of patients with esophageal body hypomotility are much higher in cohorts with abnormal pH parameters on pH monitoring than in those with normal pH studies (37.5% vs 20.0% in one study).[7] By contrast, contraction-wave abnormalities and simultaneous contractions are less common in the presence of abnormal pH testing (23.3% vs 43.5%) in patients who present with esophageal symptoms. Balloon distension studies demonstrate that contraction-wave abnormalities are associated with heightened esophageal perception, which can potentially explain how esophageal perceptive symptoms would trigger pH monitoring with suspicion of GERD in this setting.[49,50]

The most important HRM metric when manometry is performed in GERD patients is the IRP, used in excluding esophageal outflow obstruction as a mechanism for symptoms that mimic GERD.[7,33] Indeed, identification of esophageal outflow obstruction has made the most significant impact on the clinical diagnosis and management of esophageal motor disorders. The sensitivity for diagnosis of outflow obstruction is estimated at 98% using the 4-second IRP, the current standard for interrogation of LES postswallow residual pressure.[41] In addition to achalasia spectrum disorders, esophageal outflow obstruction can result from structural restriction at the EGJ from processes including esophageal stricturing, reflux and eosinophilic esophagitis, and infiltrations into the esophageal mucosa and wall.[51,52] Therefore, an abnormal IRP without obvious mucosal disease in the absence of achalasia may warrant an endoscopic ultrasonogram to rule out infiltrating disorders. Indeed, vigorous diaphragmatic crural contractions and anatomic kinking of the esophagus at the level of a hiatus hernia can also generate outflow obstruction patterns recognizable on HRM.[53]

The finding of separation between the LES and diaphragmatic crura is highly reliable in the identification of hiatus hernias. However, structural evaluations (barium studies) have higher sensitivity in the detection of hiatus hernias, and the HRM identification of these hernias at best supports the conclusion of a disrupted EGJ.[24,27] Nevertheless, it is worthwhile reporting this finding on HRM reports. HRM may play an important role in demonstrating pressure trapping within hiatus hernias, especially paraesophageal hernias, and in identifying esophageal outflow obstruction within these entities. The use of the IRP thresholds helps define outflow obstruction from a hernia, which could indicate the need for hernia repair.[41,53]

HRM is also used in the evaluation of recurrent symptoms following fundoplication. An achalasia-like pattern has been described with tight fundoplication, with LES metrics of esophageal outflow obstruction. A modest elevation in IRP is expected because of the resistance offered by the fundoplication, but a prominent elevation in comparison with preoperative values concurrent with bolus pressurization proximal to the EGJ is reported in the setting of postoperative dysphagia.[54,55] Recurrence of the hiatus hernia on HRM has been reported as a predictor of failure of fundoplication and recurrent GERD.[56] Furthermore, slippage of the fundoplication, disruption of the fundoplication with low EGJ basal pressure, and pressure trapping within a recurrent hiatus hernia may all be identified on HRM.

Presurgical Assessment of Peristaltic Function

Esophageal manometry is frequently used as part of the assessment of peristaltic function before foregut surgery, particularly antireflux surgery.[7,33] The 2 rationales for this utilization are as follows: (1) esophageal outflow obstruction, particularly achalasia, can present with chest discomfort and regurgitation, which can be erroneously diagnosed as GERD based just on symptoms; (2) extreme esophageal body hypomotility or aperistalsis could be associated with postoperative dysphagia if the fundoplication is not tailored to the degree of hypomotility.

In one of the largest studies to date assessing the value of esophageal HRM before antireflux surgery, Chan and colleagues[7] demonstrated that 2.5% of 1081 patients referred for antireflux surgery actually had esophageal outflow obstruction, either achalasia or a variant thereof, for which antireflux surgery without concurrent myotomy would have led to disastrous results. HRM has advantages over conventional manometry in that interrogation of the LES-EGJ for outflow obstruction is more accurate using the IRP metric. Furthermore, the LES can be followed proximally as the esophagus shortens, allowing recognition of the phenomenon of pseudorelaxation recorded by sensors at the plane of LES when the nonrelaxing LES has moved proximally.[41] This process ensures that the diagnosis of esophageal outflow obstruction is made with higher accuracy, ensuring less erroneous antireflux surgery for outflow obstruction.[41]

Esophageal aperistalsis from severe esophageal hypomotility can affect antireflux surgery, as a standard 360° fundoplication in this setting can result in transit symptoms. As much as 3.2% of referrals for antireflux surgery can have esophageal aperistalsis.[7] One or 2 peristaltic sequences (≥80% failure of peristalsis) was found in another 1.3%, a setting whereby confidence in a standard fundoplication is not robust. Therefore, as many as 1 in 14 patients referred for antireflux surgery could be affected by these extreme motor disorders. Limited earlier evidence suggested that partial fundoplication results in outcomes comparable with those after total 360° fundoplication, and that partial fundoplication can be performed safely in patients with severe esophageal hypomotility.[57]

Contraction-wave abnormalities and simultaneous contractions that could be associated with both perceptive and transit symptoms can be encountered in approximately one-third of patients referred for antireflux surgery.[7] These abnormalities have previously been associated with a suboptimal symptomatic response following antireflux surgery, with persisting symptoms likely from esophageal hypervigilance. The recommendation for preoperative HRM based on these data was primarily for identifying absolute contraindications for a 360° fundoplication (achalasia and its variants, aperistalsis, and severe esophageal hypomotility), and additionally for counseling patients with contraction-wave abnormalities and simultaneous contractions such that residual symptoms following fundoplication could require additional therapy with sensory neuromodulators.[7,33]

Other data suggest that tailoring of fundoplication to esophageal motility may not improve the likelihood of transit symptoms on a long-term basis. However, in the short term, the higher the degree of wrap, the more the likelihood that dysphagia develops, requiring dilation and reoperation.[58] In fact, if a 360° total fundoplication is performed in the absence of esophageal body peristalsis, the degree of resistance offered to transit results in dysphagia requiring reoperation in 38%, compared with only 0.2% following a partial fundoplication.[59] Better bolus propagation occurs through a posterior partial fundoplication than with a standard 360° fundoplication,[60] with lower dysphagia rates.[61] Others have demonstrated that preoperative dysphagia may be a better predictor of postoperative dysphagia than the motor pattern, and that both partial and total fundoplication result in similar symptomatic improvement.[61]

Taking all viewpoints into consideration, the key assessments before antireflux surgery include documentation of gastroesophageal reflux and assessment of esophageal peristaltic function, as symptoms alone are insufficient in excluding esophageal outflow obstruction and achalasia.[7,33] The fact that manometry is performed along with pH and pH-impedance monitoring ensures that peristaltic function is assessed in all patients undergoing catheter-based reflux monitoring in this setting. Modification of the surgical decision could affect as many as 7% from identification of strong contraindications for a standard 360° fundoplication, and another 23% from failure to document abnormal esophageal reflux parameters. These findings suggest a benefit in performing preoperative esophageal function testing.[7]

The issue of esophageal hypomotility needs further discussion. Although the Chicago Classification makes analysis and reporting of esophageal motor patterns uniform, the system was initially conceived for classification of abnormalities seen when patients with dysphagia were evaluated.[8] In the nondysphagia setting, hypomotility disorders are frequently encountered, especially in preoperative testing before antireflux surgery.[7,37] There is a lack of outcome data on the hypomotility designations within the Chicago Classification (small and large breaks, aperistalsis, frequently failed peristalsis) in predicting symptomatic benefit after antireflux surgery, despite data reaffirming the durability of these diagnoses over time. Taking older studies from the literature into consideration, **Table 2** describes a suggested approach to hypomotility disorders in the setting of antireflux surgery.[7] However, this is based on just 10 wet swallows, and there are new data to suggest that response to provocative measures during esophageal HRM could add further value to confidence in a standard fundoplication.

What is lacking in this context is knowledge about the natural progression (or lack thereof) of hypomotility patterns over time, especially in the setting of GERD. Although progression of hypomotility could be reasonably expected with smooth muscle fibrosis patterns seen in patients with connective tissue disorders, especially scleroderma, it is unknown whether mild or moderate hypomotility can progress. Therefore, if moderate hypomotility were to progress to aperistalsis over time, performing a standard 360° fundoplication could lead to profound transit symptoms later on.

PROVOCATIVE MANEUVERS

There has been recent interest in the incorporation of physiologic challenges during HRM to further refine the assessment of motility in GERD, particularly before antireflux surgery. Daum and colleagues[62] postulated that the diagnostic yield of HRM could improve when HRM testing is performed under an increased esophageal workload. Patients with endoscopic evidence of GERD, patients with endoscopy-negative reflux symptoms, and controls underwent HRM in the upright, seated position while undergoing both liquid and bread swallows. The proportion of patients with esophageal dysmotility on wet swallows based on previously published criteria was significantly greater in the erosive reflux group (76%) than in the control group (33%), whereas no difference existed between dysmotility during wet swallows for the erosive reflux group and the group with endoscopy-negative reflux symptoms. In terms of response to bread swallows, 62% of erosive reflux patients demonstrated esophageal dysmotility, whereas only 18% of controls demonstrated abnormal esophageal peristalsis. Increased esophageal workload with solid swallows trended toward more normal peristalsis in the erosive esophagitis group, with a significant number demonstrating normal peristalsis in the endoscopy-negative group. Failure to respond to a solid food challenge was the abnormality that best distinguished the erosive GERD group from the other groups, providing background for HRM studies involving provocative testing for improved characterization of hypomotility in GERD.[62]

These data suggest that dysphagia can be a symptom of severe GERD, and in fact dysphagia can improve after antireflux surgery.[63] By contrast, preoperative dysphagia can also predict a higher likelihood of postoperative dysphagia.[61,63] Therefore, determining whether dysphagia is related to esophageal mucosal inflammation, esophageal outflow obstruction, esophageal hypomotility, or esophageal hypervigilance (functional dysphagia) is important as part of the preoperative evaluation. A combination of endoscopy, barium studies, esophageal HRM, and pH monitoring may help make these distinctions. However, there are also reports of esophageal motor function improving following fundoplication.[60,64] Therefore, it would be useful to determine whether the esophageal smooth muscle has peristaltic reserve, and especially if an improved motor sequence can be generated on provocative testing, which would potentially indicate lesser transit symptoms following fundoplication.

A simple form of provocative testing is multiple rapid swallows (MRS), which tests the adequacy of both inhibition during the swallows themselves and contraction following the final swallow of the sequence (**Fig. 5**). Five 2-mL swallows are administered in rapid sequence, typically with not more than 3 to 4 seconds between swallows. MRS profoundly inhibits the esophageal body and LES during swallows, followed by vigorous esophageal contraction and restoration of LES tone after the final swallow.[65] This normal response to MRS necessitates intact neural pathways and an appropriate esophageal muscle response to stimulation. Shaker and colleagues[66] studied patients undergoing preoperative evaluation with HRM for antireflux surgery and normal controls, assessing late postoperative dysphagia 3 months beyond operative intervention with symptom questionnaires. Whereas augmentation of smooth muscle contraction was seen in 78.1% of controls and 63.6% of postoperative patients without late dysphagia, it was significantly less frequent in postoperative patients with late dysphagia, occurring in only 11.1%.[66] This study, therefore, is valuable in distinguishing patients more prone to developing postoperative dysphagia based

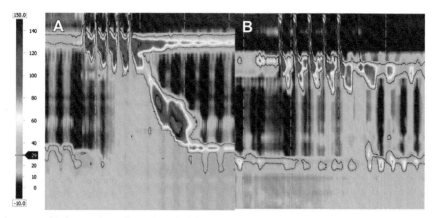

Fig. 5. Multiple rapid swallows (MRS). (*A*) Normal MRS response, with profound inhibition of esophageal body peristalsis and LES tone during the repetitive swallows, and a robust contraction sequence with reestablishment of LES tone following the last swallow of the sequence. (*B*) Lack of contraction response following MRS. This pattern was associated with a higher likelihood of late postoperative dysphagia following antireflux surgery, and may suggest lack of esophageal body contraction reserve.

on preoperative HRM. While assessment of augmentation of smooth muscle contraction may provide useful information to surgeons determining what type of antireflux surgery to offer particular patients, it may also prove useful in preoperative patient counseling.[66,67]

Thus, provocative tests are a form of stress test for the esophagus, and can reveal how the esophagus might respond if an obstruction were to be generated in the form of antireflux surgery. Esophageal peristaltic reserve is assessed by the contraction portion of the test, made evident in one study where 48% patients with esophageal hypomotility normalized their peristaltic pattern following MRS.[65] Therefore, a normal MRS response in the setting of mild or moderate hypomotility provides confidence in proceeding with a standard fundoplication. On the other hand, an absent MRS response seems to be associated with a higher likelihood of late postoperative dysphagia. Other provocative tests that have been used include free water drinking when 200 mL of water is given to the patient during HRM, solid and viscous swallows, and eating a test meal during the HRM study; these provocative tests have demonstrated usefulness in the evaluation of nonobstructive dysphagia, and research continues in determining whether there is added utility in preoperative testing before antireflux surgery.[4]

SUMMARY

HRM is an advance from standard manometry through the use of more closely spaced pressure sensors, allowing for more nuanced analysis of the esophagus and its sphincters as well as through more intuitive data displays in the form of Clouse plots. While a useful research tool for GERD in improving identification of TLESRs associated with reflux and determining deficits in EGJ barrier function contributing to reflux, HRM provides additional motor correlates for esophageal hypomotility and GERD. HRM also provides benefit in predicting which patients undergoing evaluation for antireflux surgery are more likely to develop late postoperative dysphagia while also serving a vital role in determining which patients have absolute and relative contraindications for 360° fundoplication. As familiarity with HRM increases, its role as a research and clinical tool in GERD will likely continue to expand.

REFERENCES

1. Clouse RE, Prakash C. Topographic esophageal manometry: an emerging clinical and investigative approach. Dig Dis 2000;18:64–74.
2. Soudagar AS, Sayuk GS, Gyawali CP. Learners favor high resolution esophageal manometry with better diagnostic accuracy over conventional line tracings. Gut 2012;61:798–803.
3. Arndorfer RC, Stef JJ, Dodds WJ, et al. Improved infusion system for intraluminal esophageal manometry. Gastroenterology 1977;73:23–7.
4. Gyawali CP, Bredenoord AJ, Conklin JL, et al. Evaluation of esophageal motor function in clinical practice. Neurogastroenterol Motil 2013;25:99–133.
5. Dent J. A new technique for continuous sphincter pressure measurement. Gastroenterology 1976;71:263–7.
6. Gyawali CP. High resolution manometry: the Ray Clouse legacy. Neurogastroenterol Motil 2012;24(Suppl 1):2–4.
7. Chan WW, Haroian LR, Gyawali CP. Value of preoperative esophageal function studies before laparoscopic antireflux surgery. Surg Endosc 2011;25:2943–9.
8. Bredenoord AJ, Fox M, Kahrilas PJ, et al. Chicago classification criteria of esophageal motility disorders defined in high resolution esophageal pressure topography (EPT). Neurogastroenterol Motil 2012;24(Suppl 1):57–65.
9. Vakil N, van Zanten SV, Kahrilas P, et al. The Montreal definition and classification of gastroesophageal reflux disease: a global evidence-based consensus. Am J Gastroenterol 2006;101:1900–20.
10. Dent J, El-Serag HB, Wallander MA, et al. Epidemiology of gastro-oesophageal reflux disease: a systematic review. Gut 2005;54:710–7.
11. Mainie I, Tutuian R, Shay S, et al. Acid and non-acid reflux in patients with persistent symptoms despite acid suppressive therapy: a multicenter study using combined ambulatory impedance-pH monitoring. Gut 2006;55:1398–402.
12. Zerbib F, Roman S, Ropert A, et al. Esophageal pH-impedance monitoring and symptom analysis in GERD: a study in patients off and on therapy. Am J Gastroenterol 2006;101:1956–63.
13. Holloway RH, Penagini R, Ireland AC. Criteria for objective definition of transient lower esophageal sphincter relaxation. Am J Physiol 1995;268:G128–33.
14. Holloway RH, Boeckxstaens G, Penagini R, et al. Objective definition and detection of transient lower esophageal relaxation revisited: is there room for improvement? Gastroenterology 2009;136:A527.
15. Aanen MC, Bredenoord AJ, Samsom M, et al. The gastro-oesophageal common cavity revisited. Neurogastroenterol Motil 2006;18:1056–61.
16. Frankhuisen R, Van Herwaarden MA, Scheffer RC, et al. Increased intragastric pressure gradients are involved in the occurrence of acid reflux in gastroesophageal reflux disease. Scand J Gastroenterol 2009;44:545–50.
17. Bredenoord AJ, Weusten BL, Timmer R, et al. Sleeve sensor versus high-resolution manometry for the detection of transient lower esophageal sphincter relaxations. Am J Physiol Gastrointest Liver Physiol 2005;288:G1190–4.
18. Rohof WO, Boeckxstaens GE, Hirsch DP. High resolution esophageal pressure topography is superior to conventional sleeve manometry for the detection of transient lower esophageal sphincter relaxations associated with a reflux event. Neurogastroenterol Motil 2011;23:427–32 e173.

19. Roman S, Zerbib F, Belhocine K, et al. High resolution manometry to detect transient lower oesophageal sphincter relaxations: diagnostic accuracy compared with perfused-sleeve manometry, and the definition of new detection criteria. Aliment Pharmacol Ther 2011;34:384–93.
20. Mittal RK, Karstens A, Leslie E, et al. Ambulatory high resolution manometry, lower esophageal sphincter lift and transient lower esophageal sphincter relaxation. Neurogastroenterol Motil 2012;24:40–6.
21. Pandolfino JE, Zhang Q, Ghosh SK, et al. Transient lower esophageal sphincter relaxations and reflux: mechanistic analysis using concurrent fluoroscopy and high-resolution manometry. Gastroenterology 2006;131:1725–33.
22. Fletcher J, Wirz A, Henry E, et al. Studies of acid exposure immediately above the gastro-oesophageal squamocolumnar junction: evidence of short segment reflux. Gut 2004;53:168–73.
23. Pandolfino JE, Kim H, Ghosh SK, et al. High-resolution manometry of the EGJ: an analysis of crural diaphragm function in GERD. Am J Gastroenterol 2007; 102:1056–63.
24. Kahrilas PJ, Peters JH. Evaluation of the esophagogastric junction using high resolution manometry and esophageal pressure topography. Neurogastroenterol Motil 2012;24(Suppl 1):11–9.
25. Lee YY, Whiting JG, Robertson EV, et al. Kinetics of transient hiatus hernia during transient lower esophageal sphincter relaxations and swallows in healthy subjects. Neurogastroenterol Motil 2012;24. 990-e539.
26. Lee YY, Whiting JG, Robertson EV, et al. Measuring movement and location of the gastroesophageal junction: research and clinical implications. Scand J Gastroenterol 2013;48:401–11.
27. Salvador R, Dubecz A, Polomsky M, et al. A new era in esophageal diagnostics: the image-based paradigm of high resolution manometry. J Am Coll Surg 2009; 208:1035–44.
28. Bredenoord AJ, Weusten BL, Carmagnoia S, et al. Double-peaked high pressure zone at the esophagogastric junction in controls and in patients with a hiatal hernia: a study using high resolution manometry. Dig Dis Sci 2004;49: 1128–35.
29. Khajanchee YS, Cassera MA, Swanstrom LL, et al. Diagnosis of type-1 hiatal hernia: a comparison of high resolution manometry and endoscopy. Dis Esophagus 2013;26:1–6.
30. Roman S, Kahrilas PJ, Kia L, et al. Effects of large hiatal hernias on esophageal peristalsis. Arch Surg 2012;147:352–7.
31. Roman S, Kahrilas PJ, Boris L, et al. High-resolution manometry studies are frequently imperfect but usually still interpretable. Clin Gastroenterol Hepatol 2011;9:1050–5.
32. Gyawali CP. Making the most of imperfect high resolution manometry studies. Clin Gastroenterol Hepatol 2011;9:1015–6.
33. Jobe BA, Richter JE, Hoppo T, et al. Preoperative diagnostic workup before antireflux surgery: an evidence and experience-based consensus of the esophageal diagnostic advisory panel. J Am Coll Surg 2013;217(4):586–97.
34. Leite LP, Johnston BT, Barrett J, et al. Ineffective esophageal motility (IEM): the primary finding in patients with nonspecific esophageal motility disorder. Dig Dis Sci 1997;42:1859–65.
35. Ghosh SK, Pandolfino JE, Kwiatek MA, et al. Oesophageal peristaltic transition zone defects: real but few and far between. Neurogastroenterol Motil 2008;20: 1283–90.

36. Kumar N, Porter RF, Chanin JM, et al. Analysis of intersegmental trough and proximal latency of smooth muscle contraction using high-resolution esophageal manometry. J Clin Gastroenterol 2012;46:375–81.
37. Porter RF, Kumar N, Drapekin JE, et al. Fragmented esophageal smooth muscle contraction segments on high resolution manometry: a marker of esophageal hypomotility. Neurogastroenterol Motil 2012;24:763–8 e353.
38. Bulsiewicz WJ, Kahrilas PJ, Kwiatek MA, et al. Esophageal pressure topography criteria indicative of incomplete bolus clearance: a study using high resolution impedance manometry. Am J Gastroenterol 2009;104:2721–8.
39. Ayazi S, Hagen JA, Zehetner J, et al. The value of high resolution manometry in the assessment of the resting characteristics of the lower esophageal sphincter. J Gastrointest Surg 2009;13:2113–20.
40. Nicodeme F, Lin Z, Pandolfino JE, et al. Esophagogastric junction pressure morphology: comparison between a station pull through and real time 3D HRM representation. Neurogastroenterol Motil 2013;25:e591–8.
41. Ghosh SK, Pandolfino JE, Rice J, et al. Impaired deglutitive EGJ relaxation in clinical esophageal manometry: a quantitative analysis of 400 patients and 75 controls. Am J Physiol Gastrointest Liver Physiol 2007;293:G878–85.
42. Pandolfino JE, Ghosh SK, Rice J, et al. Classifying esophageal motility by pressure topography characteristics: a study of 400 patients and 75 controls. Am J Gastroenterol 2008;103:27–37.
43. Xiao Y, Kahrilas PJ, Kwasny MJ, et al. High resolution manometry correlates of ineffective esophageal motility. Am J Gastroenterol 2012;107:1647–54.
44. Staiano A, Clouse RE. The effects of cisapride on the topography of oesophageal peristalsis. Aliment Pharmacol Ther 1996;10:875–82.
45. Kushnir VM, Gyawali CP. High resolution manometry patterns distinguish acid sensitivity in non-cardiac chest pain. Neurogastroenterol Motil 2011;23:1066–72.
46. Hoshino M, Sundaram A, Mittal SK. Role of the lower esophageal sphincter on acid exposure revisited with high resolution manometry. J Am Coll Surg 2011;213:743–50.
47. Nicodeme F, Pipa-Muniz M, Khanna K, et al. Quantifying esophagogastric junction contractility with a novel HRM topographic metric, the EGJ contractile integral: normative values and preliminary evaluation in PPI non-responders. Neurogastroenterol Motil, in press.
48. Pandolfino JE, Kahrilas PJ. AGA technical review on the clinical use of esophageal manometry. Gastroenterology 2005;128:209–24.
49. Richter JE, Barish CF, Castell DO. Abnormal sensory perception in patients with esophageal chest pain. Gastroenterology 1986;91:845–52.
50. Borjesson M, Pilhall M, Eliasson T, et al. Esophageal visceral pain sensitivity: effects of TENS and correlation with manometric findings. Dig Dis Sci 1998;43:1621–9.
51. Scherer JR, Kwiatek MA, Soper NJ, et al. Functional esophagogastric junction with intact peristalsis: a heterogenous syndrome sometimes akin to achalasia. J Gastrointest Surg 2009;13:2219–25.
52. Porter RF, Gyawali CP. Botulinum toxin injection in dysphagia syndromes with preserved esophageal peristalsis and incomplete lower esophageal sphincter relaxation. Neurogastroenterol Motil 2011;23:139–44.
53. Pandolfino JE, Kwiatek MA, Ho K, et al. Unique features of esophagogastric junction pressure topography in hiatus hernia patients with dysphagia. Surgery 2010;147:57–64.

54. Marjoux S, Roman S, Juget-Pietu F, et al. Impaired postoperative EGJ relaxation as a determinant of post laparoscopic fundoplication dysphagia: a study with high resolution manometry before and after surgery. Surg Endosc 2012;26: 3642–9.
55. Wilshire CL, Niebisch S, Watson TJ, et al. Dysphagia postfundoplication: more commonly hiatal outflow resistance than poor esophageal body motility. Surgery 2012;152:584–92.
56. Tatum RP, Soares RV, Figueredo E, et al. High resolution manometry in evaluation of factors responsible for fundoplication failure. J Am Coll Surg 2010;210: 611–7, 617–9.
57. Patti MG, De Pinto M, de Bellis M, et al. Comparison of laparoscopic total and partial fundoplication for gastroesophageal reflux. J Gastrointest Surg 1997;1: 309–14.
58. Broeders JA, Sportel IG, Jamieson GG, et al. Impact of ineffective oesophageal motility and wrap type on dysphagia after laparoscopic fundoplication. Br J Surg 2011;98:1414–21.
59. Zhu ZJ, Chen LQ, Duranceau A. Long-term result of total versus partial fundoplication after esophagomyotomy for primary esophageal motor disorders. World J Surg 2008;32:401–7.
60. Wykypiel H, Hugl B, Gadenstaetter M, et al. Laparoscopic partial posterior (Toupet) fundoplication improves esophageal bolus propagation on scintigraphy. Surg Endosc 2008;22:21–30.
61. Strate U, Emmermann A, Fibbe C, et al. Laparoscopic fundoplication: Nissen versus Toupet two-year outcome of a prospective randomized study of 200 patients regarding preoperative esophageal motility. Surg Endosc 2008;22:21–30.
62. Daum C, Sweis R, Kaufman E, et al. Failure to respond to physiologic challenge characterizes esophageal motility in erosive gastro-esophageal reflux disease. Neurogastroenterol Motil 2011;23. 517-e200.
63. Montenovo M, Tatum RP, Figueredo E, et al. Does combined multichannel intraluminal esophageal impedance and manometry predict postoperative dysphagia after laparoscopic Nissen fundoplication? Dis Esophagus 2009;22: 656–63.
64. Katada N, Moriya H, Yamashita K, et al. Laparoscopic antireflux surgery improves esophageal body motility in patients with severe reflux esophagitis. Surg Today 2013. [Epub ahead of print].
65. Fornari F, Bravi I, Penagini R, et al. Multiple rapid swallowing: a complimentary test during standard oesophageal manometry. Neurogastroenterol Motil 2009; 21. 718-e41.
66. Shaker A, Stoikes N, Drapekin J, et al. Multiple rapid swallow responses during esophageal high-resolution manometry reflect esophageal body peristaltic reserve. Am J Gastroenterol 2013;108(11):1706–12.
67. Stoikes N, Drapekin J, Kushnir V, et al. The value of multiple rapid swallows during pre-operative esophageal manometry before laparoscopic antireflux surgery. Surg Endosc 2012;26:3401–7.

Acid and Nonacid Reflux Monitoring

Dustin A. Carlson, MD, John E. Pandolfino, MD, MSCI*

KEYWORDS

- Gastroesophageal reflux disease • Esophageal reflux monitoring • pH monitoring
- Impedance • Nonacid reflux

KEY POINTS

- Esophageal reflux monitoring, although helpful in the diagnostic assessment of gastroesophageal reflux disease, has its limitations and should be used as a supporting component in the diagnosis.
- Not all reflux events cause symptoms, and not all symptoms are caused by reflux.
- Acid reflux is uncommon while on proton pump inhibitor (PPI) therapy; thus, pH monitoring without impedance may have limited usefulness if performed on patients on PPIs.
- Detection of nonacid reflux may be helpful diagnostically, however, data regarding efficacy of treatments focused on this entity are lacking.

INTRODUCTION

Gastroesophageal reflux disease (GERD), which is defined as a condition that develops when the reflux of gastric contents causes troublesome symptoms or complications, is one of the most common diagnoses made in gastroenterology and primary care clinics.[1,2] The diagnosis of GERD is often based on the presence of typical symptoms (heartburn and regurgitation) or atypical or extraesophageal symptoms, such as noncardiac chest pain, cough, sore throat, or hoarseness, and a response to acid suppressive therapy. In the absence of endoscopic evidence of GERD, or an alternative cause of symptoms, esophageal reflux monitoring can be used to assist in diagnostic evaluation.

Ambulatory esophageal reflux monitoring can be performed via several different methods. pH monitoring is available via transnasal catheter or wireless sensors and can detect reflux episodes by measuring decreases in esophageal pH. Impedance

Disclosures: Given Imaging (speaker, consultant), Astra Zeneca (speaker) (J.E. Pandolfino); none (D.A. Carlson).

Department of Medicine, Feinberg School of Medicine, Northwestern University, 676 North St Clair Street, Suite 1400, Chicago, IL 60611, USA

* Corresponding author. Division of Gastroenterology and Hepatology, Feinberg School of Medicine, Northwestern University, 676 North St Clair Street, Suite 1400, Chicago, IL 60611-2951.

E-mail address: j-pandolfino@northwestern.edu

Gastroenterol Clin N Am 43 (2014) 89–104

http://dx.doi.org/10.1016/j.gtc.2013.11.003
0889-8553/14/$ – see front matter © 2014 Elsevier Inc. All rights reserved.

pH catheters, placed transnasally into the esophagus, measure the change in electrical resistance between closely spaced electrodes and thus can determine the composition of intraesophageal contents (liquid, gas, or mixed), and measure direction of flow (antegrade or retrograde), as well as esophageal pH. Thus, pH monitors are able to measure acid reflux, which is defined as refluxed gastric contents with a pH less than 4, whereas impedance pH can detect both acid reflux and nonacid reflux, which is defined as refluxed contents with pH 4 or greater and sometimes further classified as weakly acidic (pH 4–7) and weakly alkaline (pH $\geq$7) reflux.[3] Although esophageal reflux monitoring can be a valuable tool for assessing patients with suspected GERD, each testing modality has its limitations, which need to be considered when deciding when and how to use these tests. This review covers the indications for reflux monitoring, which test to choose, including characteristics and technical details of each modality, and how to interpret results and incorporate them into clinical practice.

INDICATIONS FOR ESOPHAGEAL REFLUX MONITORING

Esophageal reflux monitoring can be used to support a diagnosis of GERD, such as before antireflux procedures, or when the diagnosis of GERD may be in question, such as when there is a lack of response to effective therapy. After an empirical trial of acid suppression therapy, generally with proton pump inhibitors (PPIs), upper endoscopy is the initial diagnostic test performed, because it can assess for complications (especially if patients show alarm symptoms, eg, dysphagia) and also confirm a diagnosis by identifying complications, such as erosive esophagitis or Barrett esophagus, which are specific, although not sensitive, features of GERD. Thus, if erosive esophagitis or Barrett esophagus are present, additional esophageal reflux testing is not necessary to diagnose GERD. In addition, endoscopy can identify an alternative diagnosis for patient symptoms, such as pill, infectious, or eosinophilic esophagitis. If an antireflux procedure is being considered, esophageal manometry is then often performed next to identify achalasia or esophageal aperistalsis; manometry can also play a role in localization of the lower esophageal sphincter (LES), which may be needed to place an esophageal reflux monitoring device. Typical indications for esophageal reflux monitoring included below.

Before Antireflux Surgery

If endoscopy is normal, which is often the case, and an antireflux procedure is being considered, esophageal reflux monitoring is then indicated. PPIs are the staple of GERD treatment and are effective in the treatment of typical GERD symptoms and healing of esophagitis.[4] Thus, a response to PPIs is often used as the confirmatory test for GERD. However, although a positive response to a PPI trial is supportive of a diagnosis of GERD and predicts a positive response to antireflux therapy, there is also potential for a placebo effect and thus false-positive results of a PPI trial test.[5,6] Therefore, even when patients have a positive response to a PPI trial, esophageal reflux monitoring should be performed in patients with endoscopy-negative (presumed) reflux disease before pursuing antireflux endoscopic or surgical interventions with their inherent procedural risks.[7–9]

PPI-Refractory GERD Symptoms

The definition of PPI-refractory GERD or PPI-nonresponsive GERD can vary, often differing in whether this includes patients who do not respond to daily PPI, or more commonly, only to patients with continued symptoms on high-dose, twice-daily PPI. Regardless of definition, refractory symptoms are the most common use for esophageal reflux monitoring. The lack of a response to high-dose PPI treatment (after confirming patient adherence and correct premeal dosing) raises several clinical possibilities: the symptoms are related to GERD, which may be either caused by breakthrough acid reflux or nonacid reflux; or, there is another explanation (not GERD, eg, functional heartburn) for the patient's continued symptoms. Reflux monitoring can be helpful to differentiate these possibilities.[4,7,8]

A special situation exists if patients develop GERD symptoms after antireflux surgery. In general, a similar diagnostic algorithm is followed as for patients with GERD without previous surgery, including a PPI trial, but with earlier use of endoscopy and imaging to assess postsurgical anatomy. If the anatomy is appropriate and an empirical trial of PPIs is ineffective, reflux monitoring, perhaps a different method than used preoperatively, again can be useful to assess for the cause of symptoms.

Noncardiac Chest Pain

Once cardiac causes have been thoroughly evaluated for and excluded, the possibility of GERD-related chest pain can be entertained. Meta-analyses have shown that GERD-related (based on abnormal pH monitoring or endoscopy) chest pain frequently responds to PPI therapy.[10,11] However, if chest pain persists or symptom cause is still unclear after a 4-week trial of PPI, esophageal reflux testing is likely the most useful test in determining the cause of the patient's chest pain.[12]

Extraesophageal GERD Symptoms

Some disagreement exists regarding the use or timing of esophageal reflux monitoring for extraesophageal GERD symptoms. GERD is frequently associated with patients who have chronic cough, laryngitis, or asthma. However, it is less clear if these observations are truly recognizing a causal relationship between GERD and these symptoms. Thus, recent guidelines recommend consideration of esophageal reflux monitoring before an empirical trial of PPIs for extraesophageal symptoms in the absence of concurrent typical GERD symptoms.[13] Others suggest that testing be considered if symptoms are refractory to PPI therapy, although testing in this scenario may carry a low yield.[8]

Assessing Effectiveness of Reflux Therapy

Reflux monitoring may also be helpful to assess the effectiveness of antisecretory therapy in patients with refractory esophagitis or stricture formation. Patients not responding to high-dose therapy may have PPI-refractory disease and may require antireflux surgery.

PERFORMANCE OF ESOPHAGEAL REFLUX MONITORING

Once the decision to pursue reflux monitoring has been made, the next step is to choose which type of device to use (**Fig. 1**): pH monitoring, either catheter-based (conventional) or wireless (Bravo pH monitoring system, Given Imaging, Yoqneam, Israel), or impedance pH. The basic equipment needed to perform any type of reflux monitoring includes a portable data logger, the sensor (pH or impedance pH), a computer, and analysis software.

There are also tests available to measure gastroduodenal or bile reflux; the most commonly referenced is the Bilitec (Medtronic Instruments, Minneapolis, MN) system. This transnasal catheter is placed with the sensor positioned at 5 cm above the proximal border of the LES, with goal test duration of 24 hours. Although bile acid reflux has been reported to cause esophageal mucosal damage and typical GERD symptoms, bile

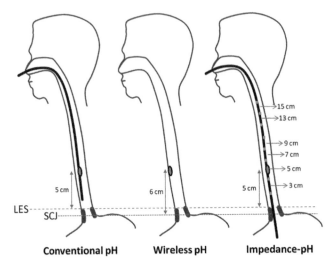

Fig. 1. Schematics and placement of reflux monitoring modalities. The pH sensor on catheter-based pH monitoring and impedance pH catheters is conventionally placed 5 cm above the proximal border of the LES, which is usually defined via manometry. Wireless pH sensors are often placed endoscopically, 6 cm above the SCJ, which corresponds to placement of catheter-based pH sensors. pH sensors are marked by pink dots. There are various commercially available impedance pH catheters with different arrangements of impedance-measuring segments, generally from 3 cm up to 17 cm from the LES, with electrodes spaced 1.5 to 2 cm. Some catheters also offer intragastric or proximal esophageal pH sensors. The pictured impedance catheter has 6 paired electrodes (*orange dots*); impedance measurements are made between the paired electrodes and marked with horizontal arrows, measurements indicate distance from the LES (proximal esophagus not to scale). Although there is no standard impedance-measuring segment arrangement, measurements should be made from at least 6 impedance-measuring segments. (*Data from* Pandolfino JE, Vela MF. Esophageal-reflux monitoring. Gastrointest Endosc 2009;69(4):917–30, 930.e1.)

reflux is commonly seen occurring with acid reflux and is also successfully treated with PPI, and thus, its use may not add much beyond standard pH monitoring.[14–17] In addition, the Bilitec system is limited by dietary restrictions during the test and a decreased sensitivity for bile reflux events associated with acid reflux with pH less than 3.5.[8,14] With impedance pH testing being able to detect nonacid reflux, the clinical usefulness for bile reflux testing is diminishing, and thus is not discussed further in this review.

To perform esophageal reflux monitoring, the sensor is first calibrated according to product-specific instructions, and the sensor is placed (further details are presented later) after a 4-hour to 8-hour fast. Regardless of which testing modality is used, several aspects of esophageal reflux monitoring are consistently recommended[4,7,8]:

- The pH sensor should be positioned 5 cm above the proximal border of the LES or 6 cm above the squamocolumnar junction (SCJ)
- Goal test duration should be at least 24 hours
- Patient instructions during the study should include:
  - Diet and activity should not be limited
  - Patients should record symptoms, meals, activities (including sleep), and position (supine, upright)
- Symptom association assessment should be used to statistically interpret studies

Various features of the reflux monitoring modalities are summarized in **Table 1.**

Table 1 Summary of esophageal reflux monitoring modalities			
	Conventional pH Monitoring	Wireless pH Monitoring	pH Impedance Monitoring
Transnasal catheter?	Yes	No	Yes
pH sensor placement	5 cm from LES	6 cm from SCJ (endoscopically)	5 cm from LES
Duration (h)	24	24–96	24
Measures	Acid reflux	Acid reflux	Acid and nonacid reflux
Interpretation	Automated	Automated	Automated, but requires manual review

Sensor Placement and Positioning

The primary basis for sensor placement at 5 cm above the proximal border of the LES is to avoid migration of the sensor into the stomach; up to 2 cm of sensor migration has been observed during swallowing, and this potential also exists with other activities.[8,18] In addition, normative values of reflux monitoring modalities have been determined with these sensor positions, and thus, accurate reproduction is needed for application of normative standards. Although wireless pH sensors, which are fixed to the esophageal wall, may offer the ability for catheter placement without risk for migration during the testing period, they are conventionally also placed 6 cm above the SCJ, because normative data are also produced for placement at this positioning.

Limitation of conventional placement location

Conventional intraesophageal placement of the pH sensor at 5 cm above the LES may limit the sensitivity of reflux monitoring by missing short-segment reflux events, because studies have shown higher esophageal acid exposures at sensor placements just above the LES (0.5 cm) or SCJ (1 cm), than at placement at 5.5 cm above the LES or 6 cm above the SCJ, respectively.[19,20] Thus, although sensitivity of reflux monitoring could be increased with placement of a wireless sensor closer to the SCJ, further study is needed to validate this technique.

Various methods can be used for localization of the LES and subsequent placement of the pH sensor. For catheter-based systems (pH or impedance pH), esophageal manometry is typically used. Wireless pH sensors can be placed either endoscopically or via transnasal or transoral deployment assembly either after endoscopic identification of the SCJ or after manometric localization of the LES. Transoral placement without sedation is possible (with a correction factor of 4 cm if using transnasal manometry to localize the LES) and is successful in more than 90% of cases.[21] Transnasal placement of the wireless pH sensor may be complicated by minor epistaxis (up to 85%) and possibly a higher insertion failure rate (8%–20% of attempts).[22,23]

Intragastric and proximal esophageal or oropharyngeal sensor placement may be of interest in specific circumstances. Intragastric pH monitoring is often performed with a sensor at 7 to 10 cm below the LES (which corresponds to the gastric fundus). Various sites for proximal esophageal or oropharyngeal sensor sites have been reported, including 15 to 20 cm above the LES, as well as various locations relative to the upper esophageal sphincter. Although there is some association of gastric pH effect on esophagitis healing, and proximal acid reflux has been associated with extraesophageal symptoms of GERD, there are sufficient limitations in regards to technical aspects, standardized normative values, and proven clinical relevance.[24] Thus, the routine use of intragastric or proximal esophageal or oropharyngeal pH sensors does not have sufficient evidence for society guidelines to recommend for or against.[7,8] Use of esophageal impedance testing, which can measure the proximal extent of reflux events, may further negate the use of proximal esophageal pH sensors, although the addition of hypopharyngeal impedance pH measurements may have a role in the assessment of patients with extraesophageal symptoms.[9,25,26]

Test Duration

Although a test duration of 24 hours or greater is recommended, there has been discussion of tests of both shorter and longer duration. In general, catheter-based tests are performed for up to 24 hours and wireless tests are performed for 48 hours. When determining test duration, factors that limit test duration, such as patient tolerance and (less so) equipment/battery longevity, are weighed against the potential advantages of longer tests, which include possible increased test sensitivity and specificity, increased symptoms for association assessment, as well as the potential for performing a single study both on and off PPI.

Patient tolerance

Patient tolerance is the primary factor limiting test duration. In studies comparing conventional catheter-based pH systems with wireless pH monitoring, patients report more nasal and throat discomfort (including more runny nose, discomfort and difficulty with swallowing, and headaches) with the catheter-based systems and more chest or esophageal discomfort (esophageal foreign body sensation or chest pain) with wireless systems.[22,27,28] Few patients (<4%) in wireless pH sensor groups required endoscopic removal of the pH probe.[27,29] Overall, patients tolerated and preferred the wireless system over the catheter-based systems.[22,27,28,30] They also reported being more active, with less change in their daily activities with wireless than catheter-based pH testing; maintenance of normal activity is important during reflux monitoring, not only to help assess esophageal components in real-life situations but also because exercise can often increase reflux events.[31]

Thus, because the primary limitation for longer duration of catheter-based studies is patient tolerability, shorter study durations have been assessed, and a range of durations (3–12 hours) and protocols have been reported (with varying inclusion of postprandial and supine periods). Studies of these shorter protocols have reported sensitivities ranging from 53% up to 97% (compared with 24-hour studies), with improved sensitivities when including both postprandial and supine periods.[32–35] Thus, if patients are unable to tolerate a complete 24-hour study protocol, some inferences may be able to be made from the shortened test data. However, limitations of these shorter duration tests, which include poor reproducibility and a diminished time frame to perform symptom association assessment, need to be accounted for, especially if a test is normal. Longer pH study durations (48–96 hours) are available with the better-tolerated wireless pH monitoring systems, which may increase test sensitivity. Wireless data receivers are capable of recording for 48 hours, but by calibrating the pH sensor simultaneously to 2 data receivers and turning the second receiver on after 48 hours, measurement for up to 96 hours is possible. Most patients are able to complete 48-hour (>85%),[27,29,36,37] and even 96-hour (41%–100%),[36–38] studies. These tests of greater than 24 hours have shown increased detection of abnormal studies, identification of day-to-day variability, increasing symptom association, and subsequently, overall improved diagnostic yield. Extending the testing period to 96 hours also allows for a single test to be completed both on (2 days) and off (2 days) PPI.[36,39]

So, although shorter catheter study duration may be an option in selective situations, it is recommended for reflux monitoring studies to be performed for at least 24 hours, keeping in mind that improved diagnostic information may become available with longer test durations.[7,8]

Comparisons of Esophageal Reflux Monitoring Modalities

Several characteristics of esophageal reflux monitoring modalities need to be considered when choosing which test to pursue. These characteristics generally include whether to use a catheter-based or wireless sensor and whether or not to use impedance testing. In addition to some differences in diagnostic yield, there are other limitations to esophageal reflux testing modalities that need to be considered.

Other limitations

When using either pH monitoring method, there is the potential to overestimate esophageal acid exposure and reflux caused by ingestion of acid foods (which may not be reported by patients). Studies using impedance are able to differentiate these events by detection of antegrade flow. In addition, pH monitoring may underestimate the number of reflux events if they occur when esophageal pH is already less than 4.0.

Neither pH nor impedance pH testing are able to measure the volume of the refluxate. In addition, although pH electrode drift is sometimes a concern, it does not seem to cause major changes in test results, regardless of sensor type and even during prolonged test durations.[36,40]

Impedance testing may be limited by difficult interpretation or missed reflux events in patients who have low baseline impedance, such as in the setting of esophagitis or Barrett esophagus.[8] However, low baseline impedance is an uncommon finding (only 1.4% reported in 1 study), and the use of reflux monitoring in these patients with endoscopic evidence of GERD may be questioned.[41] Furthermore, impedance testing is more cumbersome on the interpreting physician, because manual interpretation is required (see further discussion later).

The wireless pH sensor is also reported to cost approximately 3 to 5 times as much as the standard catheter-based pH monitor, which is another issue that should be considered when choosing between tests.[42] Additional cost may also be accrued if endoscopic placement is used or required.

The goals of any diagnostic test are to make a diagnosis and to help dictate management decisions. Herein lies potentially the greatest limitation to esophageal reflux monitoring. Although detailed discussion of specific therapies for GERD is beyond the scope of this review, a question that should be asked before pursuing esophageal reflux monitoring is how the potential results may alter future therapy. This question is pertinent in the case of nonacid reflux in which treatments for reflux inhibition, such as baclofen or antireflux surgery, may be limited by potential side effects or strong efficacy data.[43,44]

Several studies have been performed comparing the diagnostic yield of the various reflux monitoring modalities. Studies using concurrent[22] or crossover[30] measurements with wireless and catheter-based pH monitoring showed similar measurements of 24-hour esophageal acid exposure in patients tested off PPIs.

One of the primary advantages of using combined impedance pH is the ability to detect reflux episodes regardless of their pH (and then characterize reflux events as acid or nonacid). Several studies have examined the use of impedance pH both on and off PPI therapy. Although there are some minor variations among methodology, results, and conclusions in these studies, in general, they show that the addition of impedance to pH monitoring on patients both on and off PPI increases the diagnostic yield of the procedure (generally with increased symptom associations of approximately 10%–20%), although this increased yield may be more pronounced in patients actively taking PPIs.[45–50]

There are no studies comparing concurrent use of impedance pH and wireless pH monitoring; however, corresponding features, such as improved patient tolerance with a wireless system, can likely be inferred from the comparisons of wireless and catheter-based systems. Although further testing and validation are needed before clinical use, a prototype of a wireless impedance pH system has been developed and may provide exciting diagnostic advantages in the future.[51]

On or Off PPIs?

The decision to test on or off PPI can be derived from the clinical question(s) and based on the clinical scenario (**Fig. 2**). Studies have consistently shown that the total number of reflux events is similar whether on or off PPI therapy.[46,47,52,53] However, for patients off PPI, acid reflux made up most reflux events (although nonacid reflux events do sometimes occur).[46–49,54] In studies of patients on PPI, few patients had abnormal distal esophageal acid exposure,[55,56] nonacid reflux made up most of the reflux events and symptomatic reflux episodes, and acid reflux on PPIs was rare.[45–47,54] Thus, in patients on PPI, pH monitoring performed without impedance is likely to have a low yield.

When performing the test off therapy, medication should be held for at least 7 days before the test to avoid detection of rebound acid hypersecretion, although if possible, longer pretest durations of PPI abstinence should be considered, because many

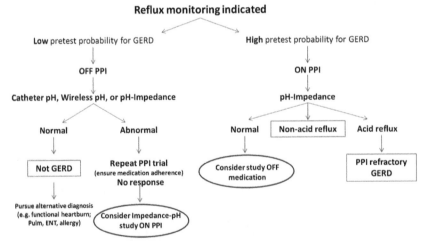

Fig. 2. Clinical use of esophageal reflux monitoring. If the pretest probability for GERD is low, such as for atypical symptoms, or if further objective evidence of GERD is needed before antireflux surgery, the test should be performed off PPI, and any modality of reflux monitoring can be used. In patients with a high pretest probability for GERD or if the clinical question stems from a patient with refractory reflux (such as whether symptoms are caused by breakthrough acid reflux or nonacid reflux), a study of PPI using combined impedance pH may be helpful. However, in some patients, especially if there remains diagnostic uncertainty after the initial test (such as a normal impedance pH test on PPI or continued symptoms on PPI after an abnormal test off PPI), an additional test performed either on or off PPI (differing from the initial test) may be helpful. ENT, ear, nose, and throat; Pulm, pulmonary. (*Adapted from* Pandolfino JE, Vela MF. Esophageal-reflux monitoring. Gastrointest Endosc 2009;69(4):917–30, 930.e1; with permission.)

patients may experience acid-related symptoms up to 4 weeks from discontinuation of PPIs.[57] In addition, 96-hour tests using wireless pH sensors may offer an option to complete tests both on and off PPI in a single test; however, the limitations of pH monitoring in patients on PPI still apply.

TEST INTERPRETATION

pH measurements from the distal esophagus are reported in terms of the percent time at abnormal pH (pH <4) and the number of reflux events (**Fig. 3**). In addition to detecting retrograde liquid reflux events, impedance studies also qualify reflux events in terms of pH: acid (pH <4) or nonacid (pH $\geq$4) (**Fig. 4**). Patient-provided data entered into the data logger can be used for symptom-reflux association analysis. Data can also be incorporated into a composite score (the Demeester score), which includes the percent of total time pH less than 4, percent upright time pH less than 4, percent supine time pH less than 4, number of reflux events, number of reflux events longer than 5 minutes, and the longest reflux event.[58] Although some studies, as well as data analysis software, report the composite score (>14.7 considered abnormal) and its various components, the percent time pH less than 4 has been described as the most useful parameter to differentiate normal from pathologic reflux.[59,60]

Although automated results from pH studies are generally reliable, this is not necessarily the case with automated impedance pH analysis software. A study comparing manual analysis with the automated scanning function of the software (Bioview Analysis, v5.0.9, Sandhill Scientific, Highland Ranch, CO) in 73 patients with GERD showed that although there was good agreement between the 2 analysis methods, the automated analysis overestimated the number of reflux episodes and had a considerable decrease in sensitivity and specificity for symptom association compared with manual analysis.[61] Thus, although the software has been updated, manual analysis of impedance pH studies, which can be tedious and time consuming, is still recommended.

Additional considerations when using study protocols with wireless pH monitors that last for 48 or more hours include which portion of the data to analyze. Sensitivity

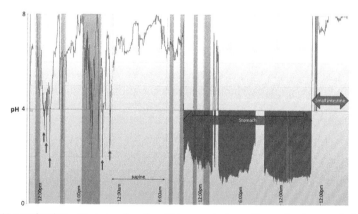

Fig. 3. pH monitoring. An example of a 48-hour wireless pH monitoring study is shown. Patient-reported meals are designated by the blue boxes; events during meals are excluded from the analysis. Acid reflux events are identified as abrupt decreases in pH (*blue arrows*). The total time pH less than 4 is measured by the automated analysis software. Notice the abrupt, prolonged pH decrease and subsequent increase in pH as the sensor detaches early (after ~19 hours) and enters the stomach and then small intestine. Early detachment occurs in less than 10% of 48-hour wireless studies. (*Data from* Refs.[27,30,64])

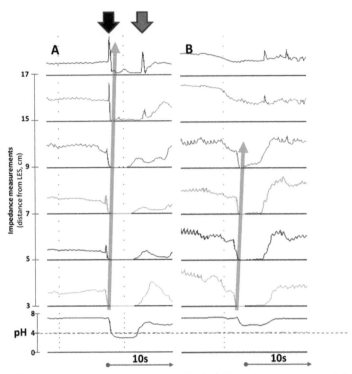

Fig. 4. Impedance tracings. Impedance detects liquid reflux events as measured decreases in impedance of more than 50% from baseline (which correlates with intraesophageal liquid) that occur in a retrograde fashion (*blue arrows*) and events are characterized based on the pH tracing as an acid (*A*) or nonacid (*B*) reflux events. Differentiation of retrograde from antegrade flow allows for exclusion of swallowed liquids. Notice that proximal extent of a reflux event can also be observed: (*A*) extends to at least 17 cm above the LES; (*B*) extends beyond 9 cm, but not to 15 cm from the LES. Intraesophageal gas (*A: purple arrow*) or mixed reflux events (*A: orange arrow*) can also be detected by observing an increase in impedance.

can be increased by use of the worst day, instead of using a single day or the entire study.[27] In addition, because studies performed with wireless pH monitors have the potential for early detachment, exceptionally abnormal study results or patient report of early loss of esophageal foreign body sensation should prompt manual review of the pH tracing to assess for evidence of early detachment (see **Fig. 3**).

Normal Values

Patient reflux monitoring study results can be compared with normal values, which are based on studies including normal, healthy patients without GERD symptoms. Normal values, which are typically represented as the 95th percentile of controls, vary depending on the type of system used, whether the study is performed on or off PPI, and sometimes, on the population tested. Commonly referenced normal values are shown in **Table 2**.[27,62–67] One of the former primary drawbacks to performing reflux monitoring studies while on PPI was the lack of normative data available for comparison. However, a recently multicenter study including 46 healthy controls off and on twice-daily PPI was performed with pH impedance to provide normal values.[67]

Table 2 Normal values	Off PPI			On Twice-Daily PPI
	pH Monitor			
	Conventional	Wireless	pH Impedance	pH Impedance
N	52	39, 48, 48	60, 72, 46	40
% Time pH <4				
Total	4.2	4.4–5.3	5.0–6.3	0.4
Upright	6.3	6.3–7.29	6.2–9.7	0.1
Supine	1.2	1.39–6.7	2.1–6.8	0.0
Number of Reflux Episodes				
Total	46.5	77–104	53–75	57
Acid	—	—	40–59	7
Weak acid	—	—	21–33	55
Weak alkaline	—	—	0–15	2

Values reflect the 95th percentiles. Ranges, when presented, indicate the highest and lowest value reported between multiple similar studies and do not reflect a combined assessment of statistical variance of the combined measures. It is apparent from these combined data that there may be some fluctuation in normal values between studies and populations.
    Data from Refs.[27,62–67]

Symptom Association Assessment

An important paradigm to consider in reflux monitoring interpretation and clinical use is that not all reflux events (acid or nonacid) cause symptoms and not all symptoms are caused by reflux events. Thus, symptom association assessment, often by using the symptom index (SI),[68] symptom sensitivity index (SSI),[69] or symptom association probability (SAP),[70] is paramount (**Table 3**) to guide an inference of causality. Symptomatic events are considered associated with reflux events if they occur within 2 minutes of each other. The SI and the SSI can be easily calculated, whereas the SAP is

Table 3 Symptom association assessment methods		Positive Test (%)
SI	(Number of symptoms with pH <4)/ (total number of symptoms)	≥50
SAP		≥95

	Reflux	
Symptoms (Sx)	+/+	-/+
	+/-	-/-

Fisher exact test

Sx + Reflux +	Sx - Reflux +
Sx + Reflux -	Sx - Reflux -

SSI	(Number of reflux episodes with symptoms)/ (number of reflux episodes)	>5

Calculation of the SI, SAP, and SSI can usually be performed by analysis software using the equations presented here.

more statistically robust and carries a more complicated computation. However, all can be generated with analysis software. In addition, symptom association can be calculated and attributed to individual symptoms (eg, heartburn, cough).

However, there are limitations to these symptom association assessments. Perhaps the largest is that they are reliant on timely patient reporting of symptoms into the data logger. Devices, such as acoustic cough monitors,[71] may be helpful for more objective symptom recording; however, this limitation persists for other purely subjective symptoms. By not accounting for the total number of reflux episodes (SI) or total number of symptoms (SSI), these measures can be misleading in patients reporting numerous or frequent symptoms, in which random temporal associations can produce false-positive results without a true symptom-reflux association. Multiple symptoms occurring during a prolonged reflux event may also not be accounted for, thus potentially producing a false-negative association assessment. Furthermore, there is some concern regarding the validity of the symptom association metrics, such that they may not consistently predict a response to treatment.[72,73] Despite their limitations, the use of symptom association assessment is important to help assess for the cause of patients' symptoms.

SUMMARY

When applied and interpreted appropriately, esophageal reflux monitoring is an important component in the armamentarium for the diagnosis of GERD. In the absence of specific endoscopic findings, a confident diagnosis of GERD based on the detection of reflux of gastric contents that causes troublesome symptoms can be challenging. Reflux monitoring can detect refluxed contents, both acid and nonacid (if impedance is incorporated), and causality of troublesome symptoms can be inferred from the application of symptom assessments. However, these tests are imperfect and certainly not the gold standard for a diagnosis of GERD. Thus an awareness and understanding of the strengths and limitations of the various available tests are crucial to their clinical use. A single test in a single clinical context (eg, on or off PPI) may not provide sufficient information to help direct management. Instead of examining results of these tests as a dichotomous normal or abnormal, it may be prudent to interpret them on a continuum when incorporating them into the overall clinical picture. Therefore, results of esophageal reflux monitoring should be interpreted within an individual clinical context and should be used to support, not solely dictate, patient management decisions.

REFERENCES

1. Vakil N, van Zanten SV, Kahrilas P, et al. The Montreal definition and classification of gastroesophageal reflux disease: a global evidence-based consensus. Am J Gastroenterol 2006;101(8):1900–20 [quiz: 1943].
2. Peery AF, Dellon ES, Lund J, et al. Burden of gastrointestinal disease in the United States: 2012 update. Gastroenterology 2012;143(5):1179–87.e1–3.
3. Sifrim D, Castell D, Dent J, et al. Gastro-oesophageal reflux monitoring: review and consensus report on detection and definitions of acid, non-acid, and gas reflux. Gut 2004;53(7):1024–31.
4. Kahrilas PJ, Shaheen NJ, Vaezi MF. American Gastroenterological Association Institute technical review on the management of gastroesophageal reflux disease. Gastroenterology 2008;135(4):1392–413.
5. Jackson PG, Gleiber MA, Askari R, et al. Predictors of outcome in 100 consecutive laparoscopic antireflux procedures. Am J Surg 2001;181(3):231–5.

6. Bytzer P, Jones R, Vakil N, et al. Limited ability of the proton-pump inhibitor test to identify patients with gastroesophageal reflux disease. Clin Gastroenterol Hepatol 2012;10(12):1360–6.

7. Pandolfino JE, Vela MF. Esophageal-reflux monitoring. Gastrointest Endosc 2009;69(4):917–30, 930.e1.

8. Hirano I, Richter JE. ACG practice guidelines: esophageal reflux testing. Am J Gastroenterol 2007;102(3):668–85.

9. Jobe BA, Richter JE, Hoppo T, et al. Preoperative diagnostic workup before anti-reflux surgery: an evidence and experience-based consensus of the esophageal diagnostic advisory panel. J Am Coll Surg 2013;217(4):586–97.

10. Cremonini F, Wise J, Moayyedi P, et al. Diagnostic and therapeutic use of proton pump inhibitors in non-cardiac chest pain: a metaanalysis. Am J Gastroenterol 2005;100(6):1226–32.

11. Kahrilas PJ, Hughes N, Howden CW. Response of unexplained chest pain to proton pump inhibitor treatment in patients with and without objective evidence of gastro-oesophageal reflux disease. Gut 2011;60(11):1473–8.

12. Hewson EG, Sinclair JW, Dalton CB, et al. Twenty-four-hour esophageal pH monitoring: the most useful test for evaluating noncardiac chest pain. Am J Med 1991;90(5):576–83.

13. Katz PO, Gerson LB, Vela MF. Guidelines for the diagnosis and management of gastroesophageal reflux disease. Am J Gastroenterol 2013;108(3):308–28 [quiz: 329].

14. Vaezi MF, Richter JE. Duodenogastroesophageal reflux and methods to monitor nonacidic reflux. Am J Med 2001;111(Suppl 8A):160S–8S.

15. Marshall RE, Anggiansah A, Owen WA, et al. The relationship between acid and bile reflux and symptoms in gastro-oesophageal reflux disease. Gut 1997;40(2):182–7.

16. Marshall RE, Anggiansah A, Manifold DK, et al. Effect of omeprazole 20 mg twice daily on duodenogastric and gastro-oesophageal bile reflux in Barrett's oesophagus. Gut 1998;43(5):603–6.

17. Netzer P, Gut A, Brundler R, et al. Influence of pantoprazole on oesophageal motility, and bile and acid reflux in patients with oesophagitis. Aliment Pharmacol Ther 2001;15(9):1375–84.

18. Aksglaede K, Funch-Jensen P, Thommesen P. Intra-esophageal pH probe movement during eating and talking. A videoradiographic study. Acta Radiol 2003;44(2):131–5.

19. Fletcher J, Wirz A, Henry E, et al. Studies of acid exposure immediately above the gastro-oesophageal squamocolumnar junction: evidence of short segment reflux. Gut 2004;53(2):168–73.

20. Pandolfino JE, Lee TJ, Schreiner MA, et al. Comparison of esophageal acid exposure at 1 cm and 6 cm above the squamocolumnar junction using the Bravo pH monitoring system. Dis Esophagus 2006;19(3):177–82.

21. Lacy BE, O'Shana T, Hynes M, et al. Safety and tolerability of transoral Bravo capsule placement after transnasal manometry using a validated conversion factor. Am J Gastroenterol 2007;102(1):24–32.

22. Wong WM, Bautista J, Dekel R, et al. Feasibility and tolerability of transnasal/peroral placement of the wireless pH capsule vs. traditional 24-h oesophageal pH monitoring–a randomized trial. Aliment Pharmacol Ther 2005;21(2):155–63.

23. Marchese M, Spada C, Iacopini F, et al. Nonendoscopic transnasal placement of a wireless capsule for esophageal pH monitoring: feasibility, safety, and efficacy of a manometry-guided procedure. Endoscopy 2006;38(8):813–8.

24. Bell NJ, Burget D, Howden CW, et al. Appropriate acid suppression for the management of gastro-oesophageal reflux disease. Digestion 1992;51(Suppl 1):59–67.

25. Hoppo T, Komatsu Y, Jobe BA. Antireflux surgery in patients with chronic cough and abnormal proximal exposure as measured by hypopharyngeal multichannel intraluminal impedance. JAMA Surg 2013;148(7):608–15.

26. Komatsu Y, Hoppo T, Jobe BA. Proximal reflux as a cause of adult-onset asthma: the case for hypopharyngeal impedance testing to improve the sensitivity of diagnosis. JAMA Surg 2013;148(1):50–8.

27. Pandolfino JE, Richter JE, Ours T, et al. Ambulatory esophageal pH monitoring using a wireless system. Am J Gastroenterol 2003;98(4):740–9.

28. Andrews CN, Sadowski DC, Lazarescu A, et al. Unsedated peroral wireless pH capsule placement vs. standard pH testing: a randomized study and cost analysis. BMC Gastroenterol 2012;12:58.

29. Ahlawat SK, Novak DJ, Williams DC, et al. Day-to-day variability in acid reflux patterns using the BRAVO pH monitoring system. J Clin Gastroenterol 2006; 40(1):20–4.

30. Wenner J, Johnsson F, Johansson J, et al. Wireless esophageal pH monitoring is better tolerated than the catheter-based technique: results from a randomized cross-over trial. Am J Gastroenterol 2007;102(2):239–45.

31. Pandolfino JE, Bianchi LK, Lee TJ, et al. Esophagogastric junction morphology predicts susceptibility to exercise-induced reflux. Am J Gastroenterol 2004; 99(8):1430–6.

32. Arora AS, Murray JA. Streamlining 24-hour pH study for GERD: use of a 3-hour postprandial test. Dig Dis Sci 2003;48(1):10–5.

33. Fink SM, McCallum RW. The role of prolonged esophageal pH monitoring in the diagnosis of gastroesophageal reflux. JAMA 1984;252(9):1160–4.

34. Grande L, Pujol A, Ros E, et al. Intraesophageal pH monitoring after breakfast + lunch in gastroesophageal reflux. J Clin Gastroenterol 1988;10(4):373–6.

35. Dhiman RK, Saraswat VA, Mishra A, et al. Inclusion of supine period in short-duration pH monitoring is essential in diagnosis of gastroesophageal reflux disease. Dig Dis Sci 1996;41(4):764–72.

36. Hirano I, Zhang Q, Pandolfino JE, et al. Four-day Bravo pH capsule monitoring with and without proton pump inhibitor therapy. Clin Gastroenterol Hepatol 2005; 3(11):1083–8.

37. Scarpulla G, Camilleri S, Galante P, et al. The impact of prolonged pH measurements on the diagnosis of gastroesophageal reflux disease: 4-day wireless pH studies. Am J Gastroenterol 2007;102(12):2642–7.

38. Calabrese C, Liguori G, Gabusi V, et al. Ninety-six-hour wireless oesophageal pH monitoring following proton pump inhibitor administration in NERD patients. Aliment Pharmacol Ther 2008;28(2):250–5.

39. Garrean CP, Zhang Q, Gonsalves N, et al. Acid reflux detection and symptom-reflux association using 4-day wireless pH recording combining 48-hour periods off and on PPI therapy. Am J Gastroenterol 2008;103(7):1631–7.

40. Hemmink GJ, Weusten BL, Oors J, et al. Ambulatory oesophageal pH monitoring: a comparison between antimony, ISFET, and glass pH electrodes. Eur J Gastroenterol Hepatol 2010;22(5):572–7.

41. Heard R, Castell J, Castell DO, et al. Characterization of patients with low baseline impedance on multichannel intraluminal impedance-pH reflux testing. J Clin Gastroenterol 2012;46(7):e55–7.

42. Roman S, Mion F, Zerbib F, et al. Wireless pH capsule–yield in clinical practice. Endoscopy 2012;44(3):270–6.

43. Mainie I, Tutuian R, Agrawal A, et al. Combined multichannel intraluminal impedance-pH monitoring to select patients with persistent gastro-oesophageal reflux for laparoscopic Nissen fundoplication. Br J Surg 2006;93(12):1483–7.
44. Vela MF, Tutuian R, Katz PO, et al. Baclofen decreases acid and non-acid post-prandial gastro-oesophageal reflux measured by combined multichannel intraluminal impedance and pH. Aliment Pharmacol Ther 2003;17(2):243–51.
45. Mainie I, Tutuian R, Shay S, et al. Acid and non-acid reflux in patients with persistent symptoms despite acid suppressive therapy: a multicentre study using combined ambulatory impedance-pH monitoring. Gut 2006;55(10):1398–402.
46. Zerbib F, Roman S, Ropert A, et al. Esophageal pH-impedance monitoring and symptom analysis in GERD: a study in patients off and on therapy. Am J Gastroenterol 2006;101(9):1956–63.
47. Hemmink GJ, Bredenoord AJ, Weusten BL, et al. Esophageal pH-impedance monitoring in patients with therapy-resistant reflux symptoms: 'on' or 'off' proton pump inhibitor? Am J Gastroenterol 2008;103(10):2446–53.
48. Savarino E, Zentilin P, Tutuian R, et al. The role of nonacid reflux in NERD: lessons learned from impedance-pH monitoring in 150 patients off therapy. Am J Gastroenterol 2008;103(11):2685–93.
49. Bredenoord AJ, Weusten BL, Timmer R, et al. Addition of esophageal impedance monitoring to pH monitoring increases the yield of symptom association analysis in patients off PPI therapy. Am J Gastroenterol 2006;101(3):453–9.
50. Karamanolis G, Kotsalidis G, Triantafyllou K, et al. Yield of combined impedance-pH monitoring for refractory reflux symptoms in clinical practice. J Neurogastroenterol Motil 2011;17(2):158–63.
51. Cao H, Rao S, Tang SJ, et al. Batteryless implantable dual-sensor capsule for esophageal reflux monitoring. Gastrointest Endosc 2013;77(4):649–53.
52. Tamhankar AP, Peters JH, Portale G, et al. Omeprazole does not reduce gastroesophageal reflux: new insights using multichannel intraluminal impedance technology. J Gastrointest Surg 2004;8(7):890–7 [discussion: 897–8].
53. Vela MF, Camacho-Lobato L, Srinivasan R, et al. Simultaneous intraesophageal impedance and pH measurement of acid and nonacid gastroesophageal reflux: effect of omeprazole. Gastroenterology 2001;120(7):1599–606.
54. Blonski W, Vela MF, Castell DO. Comparison of reflux frequency during prolonged multichannel intraluminal impedance and pH monitoring on and off acid suppression therapy. J Clin Gastroenterol 2009;43(9):816–20.
55. Charbel S, Khandwala F, Vaezi MF. The role of esophageal pH monitoring in symptomatic patients on PPI therapy. Am J Gastroenterol 2005;100(2):283–9.
56. Pritchett JM, Aslam M, Slaughter JC, et al. Efficacy of esophageal impedance/pH monitoring in patients with refractory gastroesophageal reflux disease, on and off therapy. Clin Gastroenterol Hepatol 2009;7(7):743–8.
57. Lodrup AB, Reimer C, Bytzer P. Systematic review: symptoms of rebound acid hypersecretion following proton pump inhibitor treatment. Scand J Gastroenterol 2013;48(5):515–22.
58. Johnson LF, DeMeester TR. Development of the 24-hour intraesophageal pH monitoring composite scoring system. J Clin Gastroenterol 1986;8(Suppl 1):52–8.
59. Kahrilas PJ, Quigley EM. Clinical esophageal pH recording: a technical review for practice guideline development. Gastroenterology 1996;110(6):1982–96.
60. Schindlbeck NE, Heinrich C, Konig A, et al. Optimal thresholds, sensitivity, and specificity of long-term pH-metry for the detection of gastroesophageal reflux disease. Gastroenterology 1987;93(1):85–90.

61. Roman S, Bruley des Varannes S, Pouderoux P, et al. Ambulatory 24-h oesopha-geal impedance-pH recordings: reliability of automatic analysis for gastro-oesophageal reflux assessment. Neurogastroenterol Motil 2006;18(11):978–86.

62. Johnson LF, Demeester TR. Twenty-four-hour pH monitoring of the distal esoph-agus. A quantitative measure of gastroesophageal reflux. Am J Gastroenterol 1974;62(4):325–32.

63. Ayazi S, Lipham JC, Portale G, et al. Bravo catheter-free pH monitoring: normal values, concordance, optimal diagnostic thresholds, and accuracy. Clin Gastro-enterol Hepatol 2009;7(1):60–7.

64. Wenner J, Johnsson F, Johansson J, et al. Wireless oesophageal pH monitoring: feasibility, safety and normal values in healthy subjects. Scand J Gastroenterol 2005;40(7):768–74.

65. Shay S, Tutuian R, Sifrim D, et al. Twenty-four hour ambulatory simultaneous impedance and pH monitoring: a multicenter report of normal values from 60 healthy volunteers. Am J Gastroenterol 2004;99(6):1037–43.

66. Zerbib F, des Varannes SB, Roman S, et al. Normal values and day-to-day vari-ability of 24-h ambulatory oesophageal impedance-pH monitoring in a Belgian-French cohort of healthy subjects. Aliment Pharmacol Ther 2005;22(10): 1011–21.

67. Zerbib F, Roman S, Bruley Des Varannes S, et al. Normal values of pharyngeal and esophageal 24-hour pH impedance in individuals on and off therapy and interobserver reproducibility. Clin Gastroenterol Hepatol 2013;11(4):366–72.

68. Singh S, Richter JE, Bradley LA, et al. The symptom index. Differential useful-ness in suspected acid-related complaints of heartburn and chest pain. Dig Dis Sci 1993;38(8):1402–8.

69. Breumelhof R, Smout AJ. The symptom sensitivity index: a valuable additional parameter in 24-hour esophageal pH recording. Am J Gastroenterol 1991; 86(2):160–4.

70. Weusten BL, Roelofs JM, Akkermans LM, et al. The symptom-association prob-ability: an improved method for symptom analysis of 24-hour esophageal pH data. Gastroenterology 1994;107(6):1741–5.

71. Smith JA, Decalmer S, Kelsall A, et al. Acoustic cough-reflux associations in chronic cough: potential triggers and mechanisms. Gastroenterology 2010; 139(3):754–62.

72. Watson RG, Tham TC, Johnston BT, et al. Double blind cross-over placebo controlled study of omeprazole in the treatment of patients with reflux symptoms and physiological levels of acid reflux–the "sensitive oesophagus". Gut 1997; 40(5):587–90.

73. Taghavi SA, Ghasedi M, Saberi-Firoozi M, et al. Symptom association probability and symptom sensitivity index: preferable but still suboptimal predictors of response to high dose omeprazole. Gut 2005;54(8):1067–71.

Extraesophageal Presentations of GERD: Where is the Science?

Ryan D. Madanick, MD

KEYWORDS

- Gastroesophageal reflux disease • Extraesophageal reflux
- Laryngopharyngeal reflux • Laryngitis • Chronic cough • Asthma
- Diagnostic testing

KEY POINTS

- Suspected extraesophageal manifestations of gastroesophageal reflux disease, such as asthma, chronic cough, and laryngitis, are commonly encountered in gastroenterology practices.
- Otolaryngologists and gastroenterologists commonly disagree with the underlying cause for the complaints in patients with one of the suspected extraesophageal reflux syndromes.
- The accuracy of diagnostic tests (laryngoscopy, endoscopy, and pH- or pH-impedance monitoring) for patients with suspected extraesophageal manifestations of gastroesophageal reflux disease is suboptimal.
- An empiric trial of proton pump inhibitors in patients without alarm features can help some patients, but the response to therapy can be quite variable.
- Esophageal reflux testing with pH- or pH-impedance monitoring should be reserved for patients with an inadequate response to empiric therapy.

Gastroesophageal reflux disease (GERD) affects approximately 40% of the US population.[1] Typical GERD symptoms include heartburn and acid regurgitation. However, extraesophageal manifestations of GERD, such as cough, hoarseness, and asthma, also occur. Over the last 2 decades, these entities, often called extraesophageal reflux (EER), have gained a lot of attention clinically and in the medical literature. The expense of managing patients with suspected EER has been estimated to cost over 5 times that of patients with typical GERD symptoms.[2]

In 2006 the Global Consensus Group published the "Montreal Definition and Classification of GERD," which was created via a modified Delphi process of worldwide experts.[3] Within this report, the manifestations of GERD were divided into 2 major

Disclosure: The author of this work has no relevant conflicts of interest.
Division of Gastroenterology and Hepatology, University of North Carolina School of Medicine, CB# 7080, Chapel Hill, NC 27599, USA
E-mail address: madanick@med.unc.edu

0889-8553/14/$ – see front matter © 2014 Elsevier Inc. All rights reserved.

groups of syndromes, *esophageal syndromes* and *extraesophageal syndromes*. The esophageal syndromes were classified as *symptomatic syndromes* (typical reflux syndrome and reflux-chest pain syndrome) or *syndromes with esophageal injury* (reflux esophagitis, reflux stricture, Barrett esophagus, and esophageal adenocarcinoma). The extraesophageal syndromes were divided into those with established associations (reflux-cough, reflux-laryngitis [**Box 1**], reflux-asthma, and reflux-dental erosion syndromes) and those with proposed associations (pharyngitis, sinusitis, idiopathic pulmonary fibrosis, and recurrent otitis media) (**Fig. 1**).

Four key principles regarding the extraesophageal syndromes with established associations were emphasized in this consensus classification[3]:

1. An association between GERD and the manifestations of these syndromes exists.
2. These syndromes rarely occur in isolation without concomitant manifestations of the typical esophageal syndrome.
3. These syndromes are usually multifactorial, with GERD as one of several potential aggravating factors.
4. Data supporting a significant benefit of antireflux therapy for these syndromes are weak.

These principles should guide gastroenterologists in their understanding and management of extraesophageal syndromes. This article reviews the diagnostic and therapeutic data discussing EER and provides a framework of how a gastroenterologist may play a role in the management of patients referred for such problems.

PATHOPHYSIOLOGY, OR WHAT *MIGHT* BE GOING ON?

Two general pathophysiologic mechanisms have been proposed as the reasons for which GERD may cause EER (**Fig. 2**).[4] The first mechanism occurs by direct reflux injury to the oropharyngeal or tracheobronchial structures (the "reflux" theory). This mechanism assumes that gastroesophageal refluxate breaches the protective barrier provided by the upper esophageal sphincter. The refluxate subsequently reaches

---

Box 1
Potential symptoms and complications of the reflux-laryngitis syndrome

- Hoarseness
- Dysphonia
- Sore or burning throat
- Excessive throat clearing
- Chronic cough
- Globus
- Apnea
- Laryngospasm
- Dysphagia
- Postnasal drip
- Laryngeal neoplasm

Adapted from Hom C, Vaezi MF. Extraesophageal manifestations of gastroesophageal reflux disease. Gastroenterol Clin North Am 2013;42:71–91.

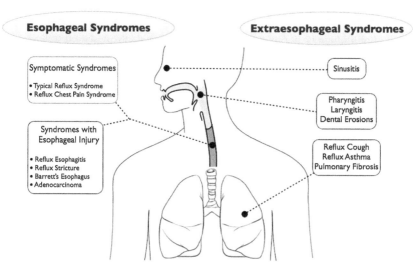

GERD is a condition that develops when reflux of stomach contents causes troublesome symptoms and/or complications

Esophageal Syndromes

Symptomatic Syndromes
• Typical Reflux Syndrome
• Reflux Chest Pain Syndrome

Syndromes with Esophageal Injury
• Reflux Esophagitis
• Reflux Stricture
• Barrett's Esophagus
• Adenocarcinoma

Extraesophageal Syndromes

Sinusitis

Pharyngitis
Laryngitis
Dental Erosions

Reflux Cough
Reflux Asthma
Pulmonary Fibrosis

Fig. 1. The Montreal classification of esophageal and extraesophageal syndromes in GERD. (*From* Hom C, Vaezi MF. Extraesophageal manifestations of gastroesophageal reflux disease. Gastroenterol Clin North Am 2013;42:72; with permission.)

Pathophysiology of Extraesophageal Manifestations

Reflux Theory

• Reflux through esophageal sphincters causing pulmonary, laryngeal, pharyngeal, or extraesophageal symptoms

• Direct contact of gastric refluxate with bronchial and laryngeal areas

Reflex Theory

• Reflux into distal esophagus stimulates vagally-mediated reflex

• Common embryonic origins between esophagus and bronchial tree

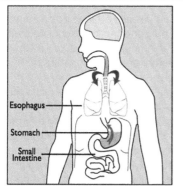

Esophagus

Stomach

Small Intestine

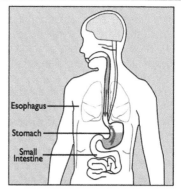

Esophagus

Stomach

Small Intestine

Fig. 2. The "reflux" and "reflex" pathophysiologic mechanisms for extraesophageal GERD. (*From* Hom C, Vaezi MF. Extraesophageal manifestations of gastroesophageal reflux disease. Gastroenterol Clin North Am 2013;42:73; with permission.)

tissues that are more susceptible than the esophagus to acid-peptic injury, such as the larynx. The second mechanism occurs when reflux stimulates the vagus nerve, leading to cough, bronchoconstriction, or other extraesophageal symptoms (the "reflex" theory). Because both the esophagus and the tracheobronchial tree derive from the embryologic foregut, they share a common innervation. Stimuli in the distal esophagus can therefore lead to respiratory symptoms via vagally mediated reflexes.[5]

DIAGNOSIS, OR HOW *MIGHT* THE ASSOCIATION BE ESTABLISHED?

Patients with suspected EER are commonly referred to gastroenterologists from primary care, otolaryngologists, and pulmonologists, often without other manifestations of GERD. The responsibility of gastroenterologists is to help the patient and referring physician understand (1) the potential contribution of GERD to the symptoms, if indeed there is any, (2) the role of testing for GERD, and (3) the likelihood that antireflux therapy will help control the patient's symptoms. However, patients often now present to gastroenterologists with the preconceived notion that GERD *is* the cause of their symptoms.[6] These cases pose a much different issue for the consulting gastroenterologist, especially when the diagnosis has come from another specialist, such as an otolaryngologist who diagnosed reflux-laryngitis, often called laryngopharyngeal reflux (LPR), based on the patient's symptoms and laryngoscopic examination.[7] Instead of providing consultation regarding the questions above, the gastroenterologist is then asked to manage or provide insight about the patient with "refractory" LPR.

Otolaryngologists often overdiagnose LPR as the cause of the laryngeal syndrome,[8] which can lead patients and their referring physicians to anchor on this diagnosis as the underlying cause. Therefore, the first step in understanding the patient's problems is to deconstruct the diagnosis into the presenting syndrome and review the diagnostic steps taken to come to such a diagnosis, the therapies provided to date, and the response to such therapies. Gastroenterologists also need to understand that they may be anchored in a preconceived notion that the patient does not have GERD. Therefore, instead of asking the question, "Does this patient have GERD?," or more importantly, "If this patient has GERD, does it explain the patient's presentation?," an alternative question may be considered, "To what degree could GERD be contributing to this patient's presentation?" A corollary to this question is, "How much could antireflux therapy help this patient?"

What is the Value of Laryngoscopy in Assessing Patients with Suspected EER?

The Reflux Finding Score is a scoring system that permits otolaryngologists to grade 8 findings at the time of laryngoscopy that are purported to be associated with LPR (**Table 1**). These findings are subglottic edema, ventricular obliteration, erythema/hyperemia, vocal fold edema, diffuse laryngeal edema, posterior commissure hypertrophy, granuloma/granulation tissue, and excessive endolaryngeal mucus.[9] However, the accuracy of laryngoscopy in the diagnosis of LPR is frequently called into question. Normal subjects without an underlying diagnosis of a laryngeal or voice disorder have a prevalence of abnormal laryngoscopic findings (at least one pathologic sign) in the range of 83% to 93%.[10–12] Abnormalities have been found more commonly during flexible laryngoscopy, usually the technique used in routine otolaryngology practice, compared with rigid laryngoscopy in the same healthy volunteer.[12] Such a high underlying prevalence of abnormal findings limits the specificity of the flexible laryngoscopic examination for diagnosing LPR. As the specificity decreases, the likelihood that a positive (abnormal) test truly represents the presence of the disease (ie, the positive predictive value) decreases. Furthermore, both inter- and intra-rater agreement of

Table 1 Reflux finding score		
Laryngoscopic Feature	**Finding**	**Score**
Subglottic edema	Absent	0
	Present	2
Ventricular obliteration	Absent	0
	Partial	2
	Complete	4
Erythema/hyperemia	Absent	0
	Arytenoids only	2
	Diffuse	4
Vocal fold edema	Absent	0
	Mild	1
	Moderate	2
	Severe	3
	Polypoid	4
Diffuse laryngeal edema	Absent	0
	Mild	1
	Moderate	2
	Severe	3
	Obstructing	4
Posterior commissure hypertrophy	Absent	0
	Mild	1
	Moderate	2
	Severe	3
	Obstructing	4
Granuloma/granulation tissue	Absent	0
	Present	2
Thick endolaryngeal mucus	Absent	0
	Present	2

Adapted from Belafsky PC, Postma GN, Koufman JA. The validity and reliability of the reflux finding score (RFS). Laryngoscope 2001;111:1313–7.

laryngoscopic findings are poor.[13,14] With such variability in laryngoscopy, its utility in confirming the diagnosis of LPR as the cause of symptoms suggestive of EER is limited.

What is the Value of Endoscopy in Assessing Patients with Suspected EER?

Endoscopic evaluation can theoretically assist in the assessment of patients with suspected EER, as a finding of esophagitis, Barrett esophagus, and/or other mucosal abnormalities could increase the likelihood that the symptoms are truly caused by GERD. However, such mucosal abnormalities are uncommonly found in patients with suspected EER. For example, in one study of 41 patients with LPR diagnosed by laryngoscopy, only 5% of patients (2/41) were found to have esophagitis while off proton-pump inhibitor (PPI) therapy for at least 16 days, although 41.5% (17/41) had hiatal hernia.[15] In another study of 32 patients with abnormal laryngoscopy suspected of having LPR, 10 patients (31%) had esophagitis, 8 of which were classified as Los Angeles (LA) grade A.[16] Similarly, in 28 patients with abnormal laryngoscopy and pathologic findings on 24-hour pH monitoring, only 5 patients (18%) had esophagitis, 4 of which were classified as LA grade A (2 also had Barrett metaplasia). Among this group of 5 patients, heartburn was present in the 3 patients with Barrett esophagus or LA grade B esophagitis.[17] On the other hand, in one retrospective study of

63 patients with esophageal adenocarcinoma, isolated LPR symptoms were more commonly documented in the record than isolated typical GER symptoms (30% vs 19%), leading the investigators to conclude that LPR symptoms could better predict the presence of esophageal adenocarcinoma.[18] However, the predictive value of isolated LPR symptoms for the presence of esophageal adenocarcinoma has not been prospectively demonstrated. At present the yield of routine upper endoscopy in patients with isolated EER is low and seems to add little value to the patient without any typical reflux symptoms or other indication for upper endoscopy.

What is the Value of Esophageal Reflux Studies in Assessing Patients with Suspected EER?

The measurement of esophageal acid exposure by ambulatory pH monitoring has long been considered a major tool in the diagnosis of GERD. The degree of esophageal mucosal injury seems to correlate with increased accuracy of pH monitoring, with decreasing sensitivity and specificity estimates in patients without macroscopic esophageal mucosal injury.[19] The recent introduction of multichannel intraluminal impedance (MII) in combination with pH monitoring (pH-MII) permits the detection of all types of refluxate, irrespective of its acidity.[20] Despite its utility in assessing the presence of GERD in patients with typical reflux syndromes, the accuracy of pH- or pH-MII testing is much more variable in confirming the diagnosis of GERD in patients presenting with a possible EER syndrome.

In a systematic review of proximal esophageal and hypopharyngeal pH monitoring for investigating the diagnosis of reflux in patients with laryngitis, up to 43% of healthy controls were found to have abnormalities in pharyngeal acid exposure. This prevalence in normal subjects was not significantly different when compared with the prevalence of abnormal pharyngeal reflux in patients with laryngitis.[21] One possibility is that nonacidic or weakly acidic reflux could explain the lack of difference between acid exposure on pH-only testing. This problem could be overcome by using pH-MII. In one study of 23 patients with presumed LPR who underwent pH-MII on high-dose PPI therapy, 52% of patients had significant nonacidic reflux and 22% had persistent breakthrough acid reflux.[22] However pH-MII monitoring is not yet accepted by all investigators because the total number of reflux events detected by pH-MII does not seem to correlate with traditional esophageal physiologic parameters.[23]

In asthma, abnormal esophageal acid exposure occurs in up to 82% of patients; however, many of these patients do not have any typical GERD symptoms.[24–26] In a systematic review of the association between GERD and asthma, Havemann and colleagues[26] found the prevalence of abnormal esophageal acid exposure in asthma patients recruited principally from asthma clinics ranged from 15% to 82%. Among asthma patients without typical symptoms of GERD, the prevalence of abnormal esophageal pH ranged from 10% to 50%.

The Dx-pH Measurement System (Respiratory Technology Corporation, San Diego, CA, USA) is a new minimally invasive transnasal device that measures pH in the posterior oropharynx.[27] This device is designed to be more sensitive to acid reflux events than traditional pH monitoring in patients with suspected LPR.[28] However outcome studies will need to be performed to assess the utility of this device among this group of patients. Furthermore, increasing sensitivity for acid in the oropharynx may lead to more false positive results. In a study of 10 patients with chronic cough who underwent simultaneous evaluation with the Dx-pH device and pH-MII, 44% (17/39) of acid "reflux" events detected by the Dx-pH device were characterized as swallows by impedance, and 38% (15/39) of events were not associated with a reflux event on pH-MII recording.[29]

Direct measurement of the association between symptoms and reflux events is another potential benefit of reflux monitoring. However the value of these measurements has recently been called into question. In a study by Kavitt and colleagues,[30] investigators used an acoustic cough monitor to assess the accuracy of patient-reported cough symptoms during pH-MII testing. They found that patients significantly underreported their cough episodes. This inaccuracy suggests that using a patient-reported symptom association measure (ie, symptom index or symptom association probability) is not likely to reflect the true association between cough and specific reflux events. With underreporting of cough, these indices are more likely to be falsely negative. However, if a patient reports a cough at a time remote from an actual cough event, the indices could be falsely positive.

TREATMENT, OR HOW WELL A THERAPEUTIC TRIAL WITH ANTIREFLUX THERAPY MIGHT HELP?
Reflux Cough Syndrome

A recent Cochrane meta-analysis that included 19 studies (13 in adults, 6 in children) concluded that there was insufficient evidence to confirm that PPI therapy is universally beneficial for reflux-related cough.[31] In 9 studies comparing PPI to placebo, prolonged PPI therapy (2–3 months) did not show statistically significant improvement over placebo in resolution of cough (odds ratio 0.46; 95% CI 0.19–1.15). Two subsequent randomized controlled trials, both using twice-daily esomeprazole (either 20 mg/dose for 8 weeks[32] or 40 mg/dose for 12 weeks[33]), have augmented the body of data refuting the utility of PPI therapy for patients with chronic cough. In the latter study, randomization was stratified based on the results of pH testing. Even within the subgroup of patients with abnormal pH testing (as defined by a DeMeester score >14.7), high-dose PPI therapy did not show statistically significant differences in the cough-related outcomes.[33]

Over the last several years, chronic sensory neuropathic cough (**Box 2**) has been used to describe an idiopathic chronic cough, often with a sensation of a tickle in the throat, neck, or sternal notch, and associated with one or more triggers.[34] In sensory neuropathic cough, the pathogenesis of the cough is related to an abnormal

---

Box 2
Potential characteristics of chronic sensory neuropathic cough

- Cough is intractable, idiopathic, and longstanding

- Cough is often preceded by tickle sensation in throat, neck, or chest

- Cough occurs spontaneously or in association with one or more triggers[a]

- Cough is usually nonproductive[b]

- Occasional severe cough attacks can last several seconds to a few minutes

- Severe cough attacks can be accompanied by rhinorrhea, vomiting, occasionally laryngospasm, syncope, or near-syncope

[a] Common triggers include talking, laughing loudly, singing, swallowing (without aspiration), yawning, inhaling cold air, changing position, or touching a specific spot on the neck.
[b] If productivity is described, it is always at the end of a severe attack, resulting from the cough instead of causing the cough.
Adapted from Bastian RW, Vaidya AM, Delsupehe KG. Sensory neuropathic cough: a common and treatable cause of chronic cough. Otolaryngol Head Neck Surg 2006;135:17–21; with permission.

intrinsic cough reflex as opposed to the specific aggravating factor such as GERD (**Fig. 3**).[35] Based on this model, medical therapy with neuromodulating medications (eg, gabapentin, pregabalin, amitriptyline) directed at improving the abnormal reflex has been used. In one study of 18 patients referred to a specialty esophageal clinical with cough and suspected EER, low-dose gabapentin (100–900 mg/day; median 100 mg/day) significantly improved cough in 12 of 17 (71%) patients.[36] The response to gabapentin did not depend on the results of the pH or pH-MII study. In a randomized double-blind placebo-controlled trial of gabapentin in 62 patients with refractory chronic cough, gabapentin significantly improved cough-specific quality of life compared with placebo (74% vs 46%; $P = .038$).[37] In this study, the dose of gabapentin was increased from 300 mg to 1800 mg over a 6-day escalation period, unless their cough symptoms were eliminated or they developed intolerable side effects, and was maintained for a 10-week period. Patients had negative investigations for GERD or negative responses to trials of antireflux therapy, although the details of the evaluation for GERD were not specified. Side effects of gabapentin occurred in 10/32 (31%) patients compared with 10% among patients in the placebo group ($P = .059$) and most commonly consisted of nausea, dizziness, and/or fatigue. Although these studies did not specifically address reflux-related cough, the premise that a neuromodulator can be effective in treating cough provides hope for patients referred to gastroenterologists for this particular problem.

Baclofen, a GABA-agonist that inhibits transient lower esophageal relaxations, has also been used to suppress cough. In patients without GERD, the antitussive effect of baclofen is proposed to be related to central and potential peripheral inhibition of the cough reflex. In a study of 20 healthy, nonsmoking volunteers, subjects were randomized to receive baclofen 10 mg orally 3 times a day for 14 days or placebo after undergoing a capsaicin cough challenge.[38] Following treatment, 6/10 (60%) subjects receiving baclofen compared with 0/10 (0%) of controls showed a significant increase in capsaicin cough threshold ($P = .005$). In a small uncontrolled investigation of patients with refractory chronic cough and GERD diagnosed by pH-MII, baclofen 20 mg 3 times daily for 8 weeks as an adjunct to PPI therapy completed or significantly improved cough in 9 patients (56%).[39]

Reflux Asthma Syndrome

The benefit of antireflux therapy in patients with suspected reflux-associated asthma is controversial, in part because of differences in outcomes used across studies and by the multifactorial nature of the pathophysiology of asthma. A Cochrane review published in 2003 examined the effect of medical or surgical antireflux therapy on asthma

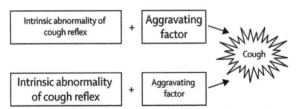

Fig. 3. Model for pathogenesis of nonasthmatic chronic cough. Chronic cough relies on the combination of a pre-existing abnormality of the cough reflex plus aggravating factors. When the aggravating factor has a small effect, such as in GERD, the benefits of treatment or removal of that factor will be smaller. (*From* Pavord ID, Chung KF. Management of chronic cough. Lancet 2008;371:1376; with permission.)

in patients diagnosed with GERD.[40] No consistent benefit of antireflux therapy was demonstrated in this meta-analysis. This review also concluded that there may be some subgroups of patients who respond to antireflux therapy, but no obvious predictors for response to therapy were identified. Several studies published since the last Cochrane review continue to cast doubt on the value of GERD symptoms, pH testing, or endoscopy, as a predictor of response to antireflux therapy.[41–45] Even though a recent meta-analysis found that PPI therapy increased morning peak expiratory flow rate, the small but statistically significant improvement (8.7 L/min; 95% CI 2.35–15.02) is not sufficient to justify the use of PPIs broadly in patients with asthma.[46] In a study of 412 adults with poorly controlled asthma and minimal to no symptoms, esomeprazole 40 mg twice daily did not improve the number of episodes of poor asthma control (2.3 vs 2.5 per year; $P = .66$) compared with placebo.[43] Similar to other investigations, 24-hour pH monitoring did not identify a subgroup of patients with an augmented response to PPI therapy. In a similar study of 306 children with poorly controlled asthma using inhaled corticosteroids and without reflux symptoms, therapy with weight-based doses of lansoprazole for 6 months did not improve asthma control or lung function compared with placebo.[47] However, use of lansoprazole was associated with a greater incidence of adverse events, including upper respiratory tract infections, sore throat, and episodes of bronchitis.

Reflux Laryngitis Syndrome

With the overdiagnosis of LPR, it should come as no surprise that the benefit of antireflux therapy in patients labeled with this diagnosis is questionable. Unfortunately the gastroenterology and otolaryngology communities do not agree on the underlying contribution of GERD in the pathophysiology of symptoms attributed to LPR.[48–50] For patients with suspected LPR based purely on symptoms and laryngoscopy, therapy with PPIs is only supported by weak scientific evidence, usually in uncontrolled investigations.[51] Furthermore impressive benefits of PPIs in LPR have not been regularly seen in randomized controlled trials. In a meta-analysis of randomized controlled trials published, the benefit of PPI therapy on symptom improvement was modest and not statistically significant (pooled risk ratio for $\geq$50% improvement in symptoms: 1.28, 95% CI 0.94–1.74).[52] Since this meta-analysis, additional randomized controlled trials have been published, some of which suggested improvement in laryngeal signs[53,54] and/or symptoms,[53] some of which have not.[55]

Some patients may indeed benefit from aggressive antireflux therapy, but identifying which patients are likely to respond remains difficult. The pretreatment presence of heartburn may increase the likelihood of an early response to PPIs, whereas higher levels of anxiety before therapy may decrease the likelihood of response.[56] The predictive value of pretherapy laryngoscopy is uncertain, as inclusion criteria for most studies of LPR require abnormal laryngeal signs. In one study, pretreatment abnormalities of the interarytenoid mucosa and true vocal folds were predictive of response to twice-daily PPI therapy.[57] Reflux testing by pH monitoring may have some value in predicting which patients will respond to antireflux therapy.[58] Most randomized placebo-controlled studies have not found any predictive value of pH studies but were underpowered to assess this parameter.[52] One recent study was designed specifically to assess the predictive value of esophagopharyngeal pH monitoring with 3 sensors (pharynx, proximal esophagus, and distal esophagus) for the response to PPIs. Among patients with no concomitant typical reflux syndrome, a positive composite pH score was strongly predictive of response to 3 months of esomeprazole 40 mg twice daily (63% vs 17%, $P = .004$).[59] The added value of impedance monitoring to traditional pH testing in predicting response to antireflux therapy is not yet well-established. In one study, abnormal pH impedance testing with a bifurcated (esophageal and laryngeal) probe predicted the successful response to medical therapy,[60] whereas in another study with 27 patients who underwent surgery for refractory extraesophageal symptoms, impedance data did not predict the response to fundoplication.[61] In patients diagnosed with LPR who present with dysphonia, treatment with a combination of PPI and voice therapy has been shown to improve symptoms better than PPI alone.[62,63] Although these patients carried a diagnosis of LPR, studies such as these support the notion that symptoms and signs often attributed to LPR can be due in part to other factors, such as vocal overuse, allergies, and environmental irritants (tobacco, alcohol).[51]

Dental Erosions (Reflux Dental Erosion Syndrome)

Dental erosion is a progressive loss of dental tissue that results from intrinsic or extrinsic acid exposures to the teeth.[64] Several sources of acid, including dietary factors, can account for dental erosions, but GERD is the major intrinsic cause of erosion. In a systematic review of the association of GERD and dental erosions, the median prevalence of dental erosion in patients with GERD was 24% and of GERD in patients with dental erosion was 32.5%.[65] Although this association is now well-established, therapy to treat GERD to prevent or stabilize dental erosions has not been greatly investigated. In one study, patients with advanced dental erosions and abnormal 24-hour esophageal pH-metry were randomized to esomeprazole 20 mg twice daily versus placebo for 3 weeks. Patients who received esomeprazole showed a significantly smaller decrease in dental enamel thickness than patients who received placebo. Although this was a small study, the results suggest that PPI can prevent progression of GERD-related dental erosions.[66]

Other Suspected Extraesophageal Conditions

Idiopathic pulmonary fibrosis (IPF) is an interstitial lung disease with a purported association with GERD. In IPF, the pathophysiologic mechanisms have focused on alveolar epithelial injury followed by abnormal tissue repair and aberrant wound healing. Chronic microaspiration due to GERD is one of the putative stimuli leading to alveolar injury.[67,68] Based on a recent systematic review, the prevalence of abnormal esophageal acid exposure is higher in patients with IPF than in the general population or in patients with other lung diseases.[68] Typical GERD symptoms do not seem to predict the presence of abnormal esophageal acid exposure in patients with IPF. In one study of 204 patients with IPF, medical (HR: 0.51; $P<.01$) or surgical (HR: 0.29; $P = .04$) antireflux therapy increased patients' survival duration.[69]

Patients with GERD often report sleep disturbances, with approximately 75% of patients who have frequent heartburn experiencing nocturnal symptoms.[70] In a large observational study, patients with severe reflux symptoms had significantly higher odds of insomnia (OR, 3.2; 95% CI, 2.7–3.7), sleeplessness (OR, 3.3; 95% CI, 2.9–3.8), and problems falling asleep (OR, 3.1; 95% CI, 2.5–3.8) than patients without reflux symptoms.[71] Sleep deprivation itself can also increase the perception of GERD-related symptoms, which may lead to a vicious cycle of increasing sleep disturbances.[72] The prevalence of GERD in patients with obstructive sleep apnea (OSA) is also higher than in controls, although the mechanisms by which OSA and GERD are associated are uncertain.[73,74] Therapy with continuous positive airway pressure (CPAP) has been found to improve esophageal acid contact time in patients with OSA,[75] but CPAP has also led to similar findings in patients with GERD but without OSA, suggesting that the effect of CPAP is not specific to OSA.[73]

Chronic postnasal drainage (PND) has been also been reported to be an extraesophageal manifestation of GERD, but the data supporting this association are limited.[76–78] In one recent study, patients with chronic PND were randomized to receive lansoprazole 30 mg twice daily or placebo for 16 weeks.[78] At the conclusion of therapy, patients receiving lansoprazole experienced significantly greater improvement in symptoms than those receiving placebo (median improvement, 50% vs 5%; $P = .006$). Neither the presence of typical GERD symptoms nor abnormal reflux testing predicted an increased likelihood of response to PPI. Although studies such as this seem to implicate GERD as an etiologic factor in PND, gastroesophageal refluxate is rarely demonstrated to reach the nasal cavity. However a gastronasal or esophageal-nasal reflex may be responsible for increasing mucus secretion and PND symptoms.[79]

SUMMARY AND FINAL RECOMMENDATIONS

Although there is no doubt that some patients have symptoms caused by EER, gastroenterologists must be cognizant that there is overdiagnosis of GERD as the major contributing factor to the syndromes (**Fig. 4**). An empiric trial of PPI therapy is an appropriate initial management step in patients without alarm signs,[4] but the absence of a response should not come as a surprise. If patients have a complete absence of response despite a prolonged course of high doses of PPI, diagnostic testing with ambulatory reflux monitoring (pH with or without impedance) can be adequately performed after cessation of the PPI therapy. A negative test in this instance should adequately rule out GERD as the cause of the syndrome. However, when patients have a concomitant typical reflux syndrome that has responded to therapy, or if their symptoms have responded partially but incompletely, the preferred testing strategy is

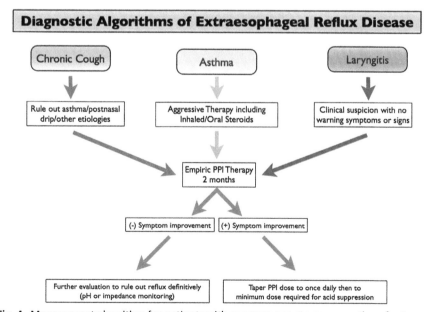

Fig. 4. Management algorithm for patients with common symptoms suggestive of extraesophageal reflux. (*From* Hom C, Vaezi MF. Extraesophageal manifestations of gastroesophageal reflux disease. Gastroenterol Clin North Am 2013;42:85; with permission.)

pH impedance while taking PPI therapy to determine if residual acid or nonacid reflux is contributing to ongoing symptoms.[80] Nonetheless, diagnostic testing, even with ambulatory reflux monitoring, is not yet sufficiently accurate to distinguish which patients truly have GERD as the cause of their syndrome and should be limited to patients with suboptimal response to PPI therapy.

REFERENCES

1. Locke GR 3rd, Talley NJ, Fett SL, et al. Prevalence and clinical spectrum of gastroesophageal reflux: a population-based study in Olmsted County, Minnesota. Gastroenterology 1997;112:1448–56.
2. Francis DO, Rymer JA, Slaughter JC, et al. High economic burden of caring for patients with suspected extraesophageal reflux. Am J Gastroenterol 2013;108:905–11.
3. Vakil N, van Zanten SV, Kahrilas P, et al. The Montreal definition and classification of gastroesophageal reflux disease: a global evidence-based consensus. Am J Gastroenterol 2006;101:1900–20.
4. Hom C, Vaezi MF. Extraesophageal manifestations of gastroesophageal reflux disease. Gastroenterol Clin North Am 2013;42:71–91.
5. Blondeau K, Sifrim D, Dupont L, et al. Reflux cough. Curr Gastroenterol Rep 2008;10:235–9.
6. Achkar E. The death of the chief complaint or how GERD replaced heartburn. Am J Gastroenterol 2006;101:1719–20.
7. Vaezi MF. Sore throat and a red hypopharynx: is it reflux? Clin Gastroenterol Hepatol 2007;5:1379–82.
8. Thomas JP, Zubiaur FM. Over-diagnosis of laryngopharyngeal reflux as the cause of hoarseness. Eur Arch Otorhinolaryngol 2013;270:995–9.
9. Belafsky PC, Postma GN, Koufman JA. The validity and reliability of the reflux finding score (RFS). Laryngoscope 2001;111:1313–7.
10. Reulbach TR, Belafsky PC, Blalock PD, et al. Occult laryngeal pathology in a community-based cohort. Otolaryngol Head Neck Surg 2001;124:448–50.
11. Hicks DM, Ours TM, Abelson TI, et al. The prevalence of hypopharynx findings associated with gastroesophageal reflux in normal volunteers. J Voice 2002;16:564–79.
12. Milstein CF, Charbel S, Hicks DM, et al. Prevalence of laryngeal irritation signs associated with reflux in asymptomatic volunteers: impact of endoscopic technique (rigid vs. flexible laryngoscope). Laryngoscope 2005;115:2256–61.
13. Branski RC, Bhattacharyya N, Shapiro J. The reliability of the assessment of endoscopic laryngeal findings associated with laryngopharyngeal reflux disease. Laryngoscope 2002;112:1019–24.
14. Eren E, Arslanoglu S, Aktas A, et al. Factors confusing the diagnosis of laryngopharyngeal reflux: the role of allergic rhinitis and inter-rater variability of laryngeal findings. Eur Arch Otorhinolaryngol 2013. [Epub ahead of print].
15. de Bortoli N, Nacci A, Savarino E, et al. How many cases of laryngopharyngeal reflux suspected by laryngoscopy are gastroesophageal reflux disease-related? World J Gastroenterol 2012;18:4363–70.
16. Qua CS, Wong CH, Gopala K, et al. Gastro-oesophageal reflux disease in chronic laryngitis: prevalence and response to acid-suppressive therapy. Aliment Pharmacol Ther 2007;25:287–95.
17. Reichel O, Issing WJ. Should patients with pH-documented laryngopharyngeal reflux routinely undergo oesophagogastroduodenoscopy? A retrospective analysis. J Laryngol Otol 2007;121:1165–9.

18. Reavis KM, Morris CD, Gopal DV, et al. Laryngopharyngeal reflux symptoms better predict the presence of esophageal adenocarcinoma than typical gastroesophageal reflux symptoms. Ann Surg 2004;239:849–56 [discussion: 856–8].
19. Kahrilas PJ, Quigley EM. Clinical esophageal pH recording: a technical review for practice guideline development. Gastroenterology 1996;110:1982–96.
20. Sifrim D, Blondeau K. Technology insight: the role of impedance testing for esophageal disorders. Nat Clin Pract Gastroenterol Hepatol 2006;3:210–9.
21. Joniau S, Bradshaw A, Esterman A, et al. Reflux and laryngitis: a systematic review. Otolaryngol Head Neck Surg 2007;136:686–92.
22. Carroll TL, Fedore LW, Aldahlawi MM. pH impedance and high-resolution manometry in laryngopharyngeal reflux disease high-dose proton pump inhibitor failures. Laryngoscope 2012;122:2473–81.
23. Kavitt RT, Yuksel ES, Slaughter JC, et al. The role of impedance monitoring in patients with extraesophageal symptoms. Laryngoscope 2013;123:2463–8.
24. Harding SM, Guzzo MR, Richter JE. 24-h esophageal pH testing in asthmatics: respiratory symptom correlation with esophageal acid events. Chest 1999;115: 654–9.
25. Harding SM, Guzzo MR, Richter JE. The prevalence of gastroesophageal reflux in asthma patients without reflux symptoms. Am J Respir Crit Care Med 2000; 162:34–9.
26. Havemann BD, Henderson CA, El-Serag HB. The association between gastro-oesophageal reflux disease and asthma: a systematic review. Gut 2007;56: 1654–64.
27. Wiener GJ, Tsukashima R, Kelly C, et al. Oropharyngeal pH monitoring for the detection of liquid and aerosolized supraesophageal gastric reflux. J Voice 2009;23:498–504.
28. Yuksel ES, Slaughter JC, Mukhtar N, et al. An oropharyngeal pH monitoring device to evaluate patients with chronic laryngitis. Neurogastroenterol Motil 2013; 25:e315–23.
29. Ummarino D, Vandermeulen L, Roosens B, et al. Gastroesophageal reflux evaluation in patients affected by chronic cough: restech versus multichannel intraluminal impedance/pH metry. Laryngoscope 2013;123:980–4.
30. Kavitt RT, Higginbotham T, Slaughter JC, et al. Symptom reports are not reliable during ambulatory reflux monitoring. Am J Gastroenterol 2012;107:1826–32.
31. Chang AB, Lasserson TJ, Gaffney J, et al. Gastro-oesophageal reflux treatment for prolonged non-specific cough in children and adults. Cochrane Database Syst Rev 2011;(1):CD004823.
32. Faruqi S, Molyneux ID, Fathi H, et al. Chronic cough and esomeprazole: a double-blind placebo-controlled parallel study. Respirology 2011;16:1150–6.
33. Shaheen NJ, Crockett SD, Bright SD, et al. Randomised clinical trial: high-dose acid suppression for chronic cough - a double-blind, placebo-controlled study. Aliment Pharmacol Ther 2011;33:225–34.
34. Bastian RW, Vaidya AM, Delsupehe KG. Sensory neuropathic cough: a common and treatable cause of chronic cough. Otolaryngol Head Neck Surg 2006;135: 17–21.
35. Pavord ID, Chung KF. Management of chronic cough. Lancet 2008;371: 1375–84.
36. Madanick RD, Sigmon L, Ferrell K, et al. Gabapentin for the treatment of chronic cough: a novel approach to treating a challenging clinical problem in gastroenterology. Am J Gastroenterol 2012;107(Suppl 1):S27–8.

37. Ryan NM, Birring SS, Gibson PG. Gabapentin for refractory chronic cough: a randomised, double-blind, placebo-controlled trial. Lancet 2012;380:1583–9.
38. Dicpinigaitis PV, Dobkin JB. Antitussive effect of the GABA-agonist baclofen. Chest 1997;111:996–9.
39. Xu XH, Yang ZM, Chen Q, et al. Therapeutic efficacy of baclofen in refractory gastroesophageal reflux-induced chronic cough. World J Gastroenterol 2013; 19:4386–92.
40. Gibson PG, Henry RL, Coughlan JL. Gastro-oesophageal reflux treatment for asthma in adults and children. Cochrane Database Syst Rev 2003;(2):CD001496.
41. Littner MR, Leung FW, Ballard ED 2nd, et al. Effects of 24 weeks of lansoprazole therapy on asthma symptoms, exacerbations, quality of life, and pulmonary function in adult asthmatic patients with acid reflux symptoms. Chest 2005; 128:1128–35.
42. Stordal K, Johannesdottir GB, Bentsen BS, et al. Acid suppression does not change respiratory symptoms in children with asthma and gastro-oesophageal reflux disease. Arch Dis Child 2005;90:956–60.
43. Mastronarde JG, Anthonisen NR, Castro M, et al. Efficacy of esomeprazole for treatment of poorly controlled asthma. N Engl J Med 2009;360:1487–99.
44. Kiljander TO, Junghard O, Beckman O, et al. Effect of esomeprazole 40 mg once or twice daily on asthma: a randomized, placebo-controlled study. Am J Respir Crit Care Med 2010;181:1042–8.
45. Aras G, Yelken K, Kanmaz D, et al. Erosive esophagitis worsens reflux signs and symptoms in asthma patients without affecting pulmonary function tests. J Asthma 2010;47:1101–5.
46. Chan WW, Chiou E, Obstein KL, et al. The efficacy of proton pump inhibitors for the treatment of asthma in adults: a meta-analysis. Arch Intern Med 2011;171: 620–9.
47. Holbrook JT, Wise RA, Gold BD, et al. Lansoprazole for children with poorly controlled asthma: a randomized controlled trial. JAMA 2012;307:373–81.
48. Vaezi MF, Hicks DM, Abelson TI, et al. Laryngeal signs and symptoms and gastroesophageal reflux disease (GERD): a critical assessment of cause and effect association. Clin Gastroenterol Hepatol 2003;1:333–44.
49. Postma GN, Amin MR. Extraesophageal reflux is still NOT the same disorder as gastroesophageal reflux. Otolaryngol Head Neck Surg 2012;146:684 [author reply: 685].
50. Randhawa PS, Nouraei S, Mansuri S, et al. Allergic laryngitis as a cause of dysphonia: a preliminary report. Logoped Phoniatr Vocol 2010;35:169–74.
51. Karkos PD, Wilson JA. Empiric treatment of laryngopharyngeal reflux with proton pump inhibitors: a systematic review. Laryngoscope 2006;116:144–8.
52. Qadeer MA, Phillips CO, Lopez AR, et al. Proton pump inhibitor therapy for suspected GERD-related chronic laryngitis: a meta-analysis of randomized controlled trials. Am J Gastroenterol 2006;101:2646–54.
53. Reichel O, Dressel H, Wiederanders K, et al. Double-blind, placebo-controlled trial with esomeprazole for symptoms and signs associated with laryngopharyngeal reflux. Otolaryngol Head Neck Surg 2008;139:414–20.
54. Lam PK, Ng ML, Cheung TK, et al. Rabeprazole is effective in treating laryngopharyngeal reflux in a randomized placebo-controlled trial. Clin Gastroenterol Hepatol 2010;8:770–6.
55. Fass R, Noelck N, Willis MR, et al. The effect of esomeprazole 20 mg twice daily on acoustic and perception parameters of the voice in laryngopharyngeal reflux. Neurogastroenterol Motil 2010;22:134–41, e44–5.

56. Siupsinskiene N, Adamonis K, Toohill RJ, et al. Predictors of response to short-term proton pump inhibitor treatment in laryngopharyngeal reflux patients. J Laryngol Otol 2008;122:1206–12.
57. Park W, Hicks DM, Khandwala F, et al. Laryngopharyngeal reflux: prospective cohort study evaluating optimal dose of proton-pump inhibitor therapy and pre-therapy predictors of response. Laryngoscope 2005;115:1230–8.
58. Williams RB, Szczesniak MM, Maclean JC, et al. Predictors of outcome in an open label, therapeutic trial of high-dose omeprazole in laryngitis. Am J Gastroenterol 2004;99:777–85.
59. Lien HC, Wang CC, Liang WM, et al. Composite pH predicts esomeprazole response in laryngopharyngeal reflux without typical reflux syndrome. Laryngoscope 2013;123:1483–9.
60. Wang AJ, Liang MJ, Jiang AY, et al. Predictors of acid suppression success in patients with chronic laryngitis. Neurogastroenterol Motil 2012;24:432–7, e210.
61. Francis DO, Goutte M, Slaughter JC, et al. Traditional reflux parameters and not impedance monitoring predict outcome after fundoplication in extraesophageal reflux. Laryngoscope 2011;121:1902–9.
62. Vashani K, Murugesh M, Hattiangadi G, et al. Effectiveness of voice therapy in reflux-related voice disorders. Dis Esophagus 2010;23:27–32.
63. Park JO, Shim MR, Hwang YS, et al. Combination of voice therapy and antireflux therapy rapidly recovers voice-related symptoms in laryngopharyngeal reflux patients. Otolaryngol Head Neck Surg 2012;146:92–7.
64. Almeida e Silva JS, Baratieri LN, Araujo E, et al. Dental erosion: understanding this pervasive condition. J Esthet Restor Dent 2011;23:205–16.
65. Pace F, Pallotta S, Tonini M, et al. Systematic review: gastro-oesophageal reflux disease and dental lesions. Aliment Pharmacol Ther 2008;27:1179–86.
66. Wilder-Smith CH, Wilder-Smith P, Kawakami-Wong H, et al. Quantification of dental erosions in patients with GERD using optical coherence tomography before and after double-blind, randomized treatment with esomeprazole or placebo. Am J Gastroenterol 2009;104:2788–95.
67. Fahim A, Crooks M, Hart SP. Gastroesophageal reflux and idiopathic pulmonary fibrosis: a review. Pulm Med 2011;2011:634613.
68. Hershcovici T, Jha LK, Johnson T, et al. Systematic review: the relationship between interstitial lung diseases and gastro-oesophageal reflux disease. Aliment Pharmacol Ther 2011;34:1295–305.
69. Lee JS, Ryu JH, Elicker BM, et al. Gastroesophageal reflux therapy is associated with longer survival in patients with idiopathic pulmonary fibrosis. Am J Respir Crit Care Med 2011;184:1390–4.
70. Fujiwara Y, Arakawa T, Fass R. Gastroesophageal reflux disease and sleep. Gastroenterol Clin North Am 2013;42:57–70.
71. Jansson C, Nordenstedt H, Wallander MA, et al. A population-based study showing an association between gastroesophageal reflux disease and sleep problems. Clin Gastroenterol Hepatol 2009;7:960–5.
72. Schey R, Dickman R, Parthasarathy S, et al. Sleep deprivation is hyperalgesic in patients with gastroesophageal reflux disease. Gastroenterology 2007;133:1787–95.
73. Ing AJ, Ngu MC, Breslin AB. Obstructive sleep apnea and gastroesophageal reflux. Am J Med 2000;108(Suppl 4a):120S–5S.
74. Kuribayashi S, Kusano M, Kawamura O, et al. Mechanism of gastroesophageal reflux in patients with obstructive sleep apnea syndrome. Neurogastroenterol Motil 2010;22:611.e172.

75. Tawk M, Goodrich S, Kinasewitz G, et al. The effect of 1 week of continuous positive airway pressure treatment in obstructive sleep apnea patients with concomitant gastroesophageal reflux. Chest 2006;130:1003–8.

76. Wise SK, Wise JC, DelGaudio JM. Association of nasopharyngeal and laryngopharyngeal reflux with postnasal drip symptomatology in patients with and without rhinosinusitis. Am J Rhinol 2006;20:283–9.

77. Pawar S, Lim HJ, Gill M, et al. Treatment of postnasal drip with proton pump inhibitors: a prospective, randomized, placebo-controlled study. Am J Rhinol 2007;21:695–701.

78. Vaezi MF, Hagaman DD, Slaughter JC, et al. Proton pump inhibitor therapy improves symptoms in postnasal drainage. Gastroenterology 2010;139:1887–93.

79. Wong IW, Rees G, Greiff L, et al. Gastroesophageal reflux disease and chronic sinusitis: in search of an esophageal-nasal reflex. Am J Rhinol Allergy 2010;24:255–9.

80. Pandolfino JE, Vela MF. Esophageal-reflux monitoring. Gastrointest Endosc 2009;69:917–30, 930.e1.

Medical Treatments of GERD
The Old and New

Marcelo F. Vela, MD, MSCR

KEYWORDS

- Gastroesophageal reflux • Proton pump inhibitors
- Transient lower esophageal sphincter relaxation inhibitors • Prokinetics
- Esophageal mucosal repair • Visceral analgesia

KEY POINTS

- The mainstay of pharmacologic therapy for GERD is gastric acid suppression with PPIs, with no major differences among the available PPIs for healing of erosive esophagitis and achieving symptom control.
- PPIs are superior to H2RAs for healing of erosive esophagitis and achieving symptom control.
- TLESR inhibitors have been shown to reduce reflux episodes and symptoms, but at the present time only the GABA-B agonist baclofen is available for this purpose because development of other compounds was stopped due to low efficacy or side effects.
- Esophageal defense mechanisms can be augmented by improving esophageal clearance with prokinetics but this approach is limited by low efficacy and side effects; alternatively, epithelial repair can be enhanced with novel agents such as rebamipide, but data on this form of therapy are very limited.
- Targeting esophageal sensation as a means to treat GERD symptoms may be possible by esophageal mucosal nociceptor blockade or through modulation of afferent signals and their cortical interpretation using compounds such as TRPV1 nociceptor antagonists or antidepressants, or by cognitive techniques like hypnotherapy; as with other interventions, data are limited.

INTRODUCTION

Gastroesophageal reflux disease (GERD) is a very common clinical problem. Heartburn is experienced on a weekly basis by nearly 20% of the US population.[1] GERD has become the most frequent gastroenterological outpatient diagnosis as well as the most common indication for upper endoscopy in the United States.[2] Medical treatment of this condition is primarily based on gastric acid suppression by agents such as proton pump inhibitors (PPIs). These medications are often prescribed empirically to

Division of Gastroenterology and Hepatology, Michael E. DeBakey VA Medical Center, Baylor College of Medicine, 2002 Holcombe Boulevard, Houston, TX 77030, USA
E-mail address: mvela@bcm.edu

Gastroenterol Clin N Am 43 (2014) 121–133
http://dx.doi.org/10.1016/j.gtc.2013.12.001
0889-8553/14/$ – see front matter © 2014 Elsevier Inc. All rights reserved.

treat symptoms that are attributed to reflux. Given the high prevalence of GERD, PPI sales in the United States totaled \$13.6 billion in 2009.[3] Although these medications are often effective, up to one-third of patients may have insufficient symptomatic relief despite their use.[4] Thus, a very important clinical challenge in the current era of rising GERD prevalence[5] and very frequent PPI use is the large number of patients in whom symptoms persist despite this form of therapy,[6] which has created a need for alternative treatment approaches. As with any disease state, the pathophysiology of the disorder provides specific therapeutic targets. In this article, existing as well as new and evolving approaches to treating GERD are discussed, focusing on pathophysiology-based therapeutic targets.

A PATHOPHYSIOLOGY-BASED APPROACH TO THE MEDICAL TREATMENT OF GERD

In a generally accepted pathophysiological model of GERD,[7,8] reflux of gastric contents into the esophagus occurs as a result of the interplay among different factors in the upper gastrointestinal tract. Potentially harmful agents to the esophageal mucosa include gastric (acid and pepsin) or duodenal (bile acids and trypsin) secretions. To prevent movement of these harmful gastroduodenal contents into the esophagus, the lower esophageal sphincter (LES), in concert with the crural diaphragm, forms a barrier at the esophagogastric junction. If this barrier is breached and the esophageal mucosa is exposed to the damaging gastroduodenal agents, mucosal protection occurs through esophageal clearance facilitated by peristalsis, and by epithelial defense and repair mechanisms. The pathophysiological sequence of events leading to GERD manifestations may include (1) frequent failure of the antireflux barrier due to transient LES relaxations, a hypotensive LES, or anatomic disruption of the esophagogastric junction (ie, hiatus hernia); (2) the occurrence of reflux episodes with specific physicochemical characteristics, such as liquid/gas composition, acidity, and proximal extension of refluxate in the esophagus[9]; (3) macroscopic or microscopic loss of esophageal mucosal integrity due to exposure to gastric contents that is frequent or severe enough to overwhelm the esophageal defense mechanisms[10]; (4) activation of esophageal mucosa nociceptors[11]; (5) triggering of afferent signaling pathways[12]; (6) cortical processing of these signals leading to the perception of heartburn or other symptoms of GERD.[13]

In terms of pharmacologic approaches to the treatment of GERD, one can intervene in any of the steps in the above sequence (**Table 1**) through (1) altering gastric contents by neutralization of acid; (2) augmentation of the antireflux barrier; (3) enhancement of mucosal defense mechanisms (improving esophageal clearance and epithelial defense/repair); (4) blocking esophageal nociceptors; (5) modulation of afferent signals and their interpretation in the brain cortex.

Neutralization of Gastric Contents

Neutralization of gastric acid has been a mainstay of medical therapy for GERD for many years and can be achieved through antacids, histamine-2 receptor antagonists (H2RAs), or PPIs.

Antacids are not antisecretory agents; they neutralize acid that has been secreted into the stomach but they do not block the acid secreting proton pumps. Antacids are primarily used for relief of mild infrequent symptoms[14]; they can also be used for occasional breakthrough symptoms in patients taking PPIs. Options for antisecretory therapy include H2RAs and PPIs. H2RAs competitively block histamine-stimulated acid secretion. The available H2RAs (famotidine, ranitidine, nizatidine, cimetidine) are equivalent in their ability to suppress gastric acid secretion and control

Table 1
Potential therapeutic interventions for GERD based on their corresponding pathophysiological mechanism

Pathophysiological Mechanism	Therapeutic Intervention
Gastric acid is harmful to the esophageal mucosa if reflux occurs	Gastric acid neutralization • Antacids • Histamine-2 receptor antagonists • Proton pump inhibitors
Failure of the antireflux barrier leads to reflux episodes	TLESR inhibitors • GABA-B agonists • mGluR5 antagonists • Other: cannabinoid receptor agonists, CCK antagonists
Esophageal defense mechanisms are overwhelmed as a result of frequent reflux, leading to loss of mucosal integrity	Prokinetics (enhance peristalsis and clearance) • Metoclopramide, domperidone, itopride, mosapride Enhance mucosal defense • Rebamipide
Activation of nociceptors in esophageal mucosa	TRPV1 receptor antagonists • AZD1386
Firing of afferent signals, interpretation of these signals in the brain cortex resulting in perception of symptoms	Antidepressants • SSRIs, others Cognitive approaches • Acupuncture • Hypnosis • Johrei

Abbreviation: SSRIs, selective serotonin reuptake inhibitors.

symptoms.[15] PPIs are more potent than H2RAs because they block the final common pathway for acid secretion by covalently binding to the proton pump, thus blocking the $H^+/K^+ATPase$ exchange pathway.

Comparative effectiveness of H2RAs versus PPIs
Although H2RAs have been shown to be superior to placebo for healing erosive esophagitis (EE) and controlling heartburn, PPIs are more effective than H2RAs and have become the therapy of choice for healing esophagitis and providing symptomatic relief. That PPIs are superior to H2RAs has been well established for quite some time and thus the studies evaluating this issue are several years old. In a 1997 meta-analysis, the mean (±SD) overall proportion of healed EE irrespective of drug dose or treatment duration was highest with PPIs (84% ± 11%) versus H2RAs (52% ± 17%), or placebo (28% ± 16%).[16] The mean proportion of patients who became heartburn-free was also higher with PPIs (77.4% ± 10.4%) versus H2RAs (47.6% ± 15.5%), and PPIs provided faster, more complete heartburn relief (11.5%/wk) versus H2RAs (6.4%/wk).

More than a decade ago, a few studies suggested that H2RAs may be useful for night-time acid suppression in patients who experienced nocturnal reflux symptoms despite taking a twice-daily PPI.[17] However, higher quality studies with prolonged follow-up later on showed tachyphylaxis for this effect of H2RAs.[18] Therefore, although they can be used intermittently on an as-needed basis for breakthrough nocturnal symptoms, a standing nighttime dose of H2RAs cannot be recommended for these patients.

Comparative effectiveness of different PPIs

Seven PPIs are currently in use in the United States; 3 are available over the counter (omeprazole, lansoprazole, and omeprazole-sodium bicarbonate) and the other 4 can only be obtained by prescription (rabeprazole, pantoprazole, esomeprazole, and dexlansoprazole). A 2006 meta-analysis compared the efficacy of esomeprazole versus 3 other PPIs (omeprazole, lansoprazole, and pantoprazole) in patients with EE.[19] The meta-analysis, which included 15,316 patients in 10 studies, found that at 8 weeks, there was a 5% relative increase (relative risk [RR], 1.05; 95% confidence interval [CI] 1.02–1.08) in the probability of healing of EE with esomeprazole, yielding an absolute risk reduction of 4% and number needed to treat of 25. The calculated number needed to treat by Los Angeles grade of EE (LA grades A–D) were 50, 33, 14, and 8, respectively. Esomeprazole conferred an 8% relative increase (RR, 1.08; 95% CI 1.05–1.11) in the probability of GERD symptom relief at 4 weeks. Although esomeprazole appeared to confer a statistically significant improvement, there was only modest clinical benefit in 8-week healing of esophagitis and symptom relief in all-comers with EE. The clinical benefit appeared negligible in less severe erosive disease, but may be of importance in more severe disease. However, only one-third of GERD patients are found to have esophagitis and when present it is predominantly mild (LA grades A and B).

Comparative trial data for the more recently available PPIs (omeprazole-sodium bicarbonate and dexlansoprazole) are very limited; there are no major clinical advantages with these medications. Omeprazole-sodium bicarbonate, an immediate-release PPI, was found to be superior to pantoprazole for control of nocturnal gastric pH when each was administered at bedtime,[20] but this was a measurement of intragastric (not esophageal) pH, and whether this effect leads to better symptom control has not been studied. Dexlansoprazole, a dual delayed release PPI that became available in 2009, was found to be superior to lansoprazole for healing of EE in one trial, and noninferior in another; these studies showed no difference in control of heartburn for dexlansoprazole compared with lansoprazole.[21]

Although one can conclude that symptom relief is overall equivalent for all PPIs, switching to a different PPI for patients with incomplete symptom relief is a very common clinical practice, based on the possibility of intrasubject variability in response to different PPIs. Increasing from once-daily to twice-daily dosing to improve symptom relief is also commonly done in the clinical arena. However, there are only limited data to support these practices. A randomized controlled trial in patients with persistent GERD symptoms despite a single-daily dose of PPI showed that increasing lansoprazole to twice daily or switching therapy to esomeprazole once daily both resulted in symptomatic improvement in roughly 20% of patients, without a clear advantage for either strategy.[22] Similarly, another randomized trial found that increasing lansoprazole to twice daily was as effective as changing it to omeprazole once daily in patients with incomplete response to once-daily lansoprazole.[23] There are no available data evaluating the effect of switching PPIs more than once.

Comparative effectiveness of PPIs versus anti-reflux surgery

Laparoscopic anti-reflux surgery (LARS) is a well-established treatment for GERD, with high-quality trials supporting its efficacy in patients with esophagitis as well as those with abnormal distal esophageal acid exposure on ambulatory reflux monitoring.[24] A recent, multicenter randomized clinical trial assessed symptomatic remission after a 5-year follow-up in 180 patients treated with laparoscopic fundoplication versus 192 treated with esomeprazole.[25] All patients had EE or abnormal pH at baseline, and they had all responded to esomeprazole in a 3-month run-in period.

Estimated remission rates at 5 years were 92% (95% CI 89%–96%) in the esomeprazole group and 85% (95% CI 81%–90%) in the LARS group (log-rank $P = .048$). The difference between groups was no longer statistically significant following best-case scenario modeling of the effects of study dropout. The prevalence and severity of heartburn at 5 years were similar for the esomeprazole and LARS groups (16% and 8%, $P<.14$); regurgitation was more frequent with esomeprazole (13% and 2%, $P<.001$), but other symptoms were more common after fundoplication: 5% and 11% for dysphagia ($P<.001$), 28% and 40% for bloating ($P<.001$), and 40% and 57% for flatulence ($P<.001$). Thus, this high-quality trial with long-term follow-up showed that with contemporary antireflux therapy for GERD, either by pharmacologic acid suppression with esomeprazole or by laparoscopic fundoplication, most patients achieve and remain in remission at 5 years.

Potassium-competitive acid blockers
In contrast to PPIs, which bind to proton pumps in an irreversible fashion, potassium-competitive acid blockers (PCABs) inhibit $H^+/K^+ATPase$ in a competitive and reversible manner. Additional differences from PPIs include a higher concentration in the parietal cell compared with plasma, and a peak effect after the first dose rather than after repeated dosing.[26] Despite these potential pharmacokinetic and pharmacodynamic advantages, none of these agents have made it to the clinical arena because of side effects or a lack of superiority when compared with PPIs. For instance, the PCAB AZD8065 was found to have similar efficacy for healing EE and controlling heartburn when compared with omeprazole.[27] Whether PCABs with greater effectiveness than PPIs along with an acceptable side effect profile will become available in the future remains to be seen.

Augmentation of the Antireflux Barrier Function
All of the pharmacologic agents that work by neutralizing gastric acid do not prevent gastroesophageal reflux from occurring; they simply alter the gastric contents, rendering them less harmful to the esophageal mucosa. Although acid suppression is an effective therapy for symptom control in many patients, up to one-third will continue to experience uncomfortable symptoms despite acid suppression with PPIs. In some of these patients, the persistent symptoms are due to ongoing reflux of either acid or nonacid (ie, with a pH above 4.0, also termed weakly acidic) material. An early study in heartburn patients that underwent impedance-pH monitoring before and after 7 days of omeprazole found that PPI therapy did not achieve a significant reduction in the total number of reflux episodes (acid and nonacid reflux combined), causing instead a change in the ratio of acid to nonacid reflux.[28] After PPI therapy the percentage of acid reflux decreased from 45% to 3%, while nonacid reflux increased from 55% to 97%. Heartburn was more commonly linked to acid reflux but was also induced by nonacid reflux, and regurgitation was unchanged by acid suppression because it was frequently caused by nonacid reflux in the treated state. The observation that nonacid reflux can cause symptoms that are indistinguishable from those that are caused by acid has been corroborated by subsequent studies.[9,29] Furthermore, a systematic review that quantified acid and nonacid reflux in studies of GERD patients taking a PPI found that weakly acidic reflux underlies most reflux episodes in these patients and is the main cause of persistent symptoms despite PPI therapy.[30]

  One approach for the management of acid or nonacid reflux in these patients is to focus on augmenting the function of the antireflux barrier and this can be accomplished through fundoplication,[31] or by pharmacologic inhibition of transient lower esophageal sphincter relaxations (TLESRs). TLESRs are not induced by swallowing and instead occur through a vago-vagal reflex that is triggered by gastric distension.[32] Several neurotransmitters and receptors have been found to be involved in the modulation of TLESRs, including nitric oxide, opioids, cholecystokinin (CCK), muscarinic receptors, and cannabinoid receptors; among these, γ-aminobutyric acid (GABA) and glutamate may be the dominant neurotransmitters in this signaling pathway.[33,34]

GABA-B agonists

The GABA-B agonist baclofen has been available for many years for the treatment of spasticity. More recently, this agent was found to reduce TLESRs and reflux episodes in humans.[35] Baclofen has also been shown to decrease the number of postprandial acid and nonacid reflux events,[36] nocturnal reflux activity,[37] and duodenogastric reflux as detected by monitoring for bile reflux.[38] Given the limited treatment options for GERD symptoms refractory to PPIs, a trial of baclofen at a dosage of 5 to 20 mg TID can be considered in patients with objective documentation of continued symptomatic reflux despite optimal PPI therapy, but there are no long-term data evaluating the efficacy of baclofen in GERD. Furthermore, its use is limited by frequent side effects, including nausea, somnolence, dizziness, and fatigue. Furthermore, baclofen is not US Food and Drug Administration–approved for the treatment of GERD.

Newer GABA-B agonists have been developed with the aim of reducing TLESRs with fewer side effects. Unfortunately, development has been stopped because of insufficient efficacy or side effects. The GABA-B agonist lesogaberan was found to decrease TLESRs and reflux episodes in healthy subjects,[39] but a randomized, double-blind, control trial evaluating its use as adjunct therapy to PPIs in patients with refractory symptoms found only modest, albeit statistically significant, clinical benefit[40] and further development was therefore halted. Arbaclofen placarbil, a pro-drug of the pharmacologically active R-isomer of baclofen, was shown to reduce reflux episodes in GERD patients.[41] However, further development was stopped after a subsequent randomized, double-blind, placebo-controlled trial showed that arbaclofen was not superior to placebo in reducing heartburn events over 4 weeks.[42] Thus, the only available GABA-B agonist at the present time continues to be baclofen.

Metabotropic glutamate receptor-5 antagonists

Peripherally located metabotropic glutamate receptors have been associated with control of TLESRs by modulation of the mechanosensitivity of vagal afferents. The negative allosteric modulator of metabotropic glutamate receptor-5 (mGluR5) ADX10059 was found to reduce TLESRs and esophageal acid exposure in a proof-of-concept study.[43] However, development of this medication was discontinued later on because of hepatotoxicity. More recently, AZD2066, another mGluR5 antagonist, was found to decrease TLESRs and reflux episodes in healthy subjects without causing serious adverse events,[44] but there are no other trials available.

Other TLESR inhibitors

The cannabinoid receptor agonists, dronabinol[45] and rimonabant,[46] have been shown to reduce postprandial TLESRs; however, these compounds were deemed unsuitable for further trials because of side effects, mainly nausea and vomiting. Another potential therapeutic target in this arena is CCK. Although the CCK antagonist loxiglumide was found to reduce TLESRs, the effect on postprandial reflux was only modest and further development was not pursued.[47]

Enhancement of Mucosal Defense and Repair Mechanisms

Pharmacologic enhancement of the esophageal defense mechanisms can theoretically be achieved by two approaches. One is to improve esophageal clearance of refluxate through augmentation of peristalsis. Another alternative is to enhance epithelial repair mechanisms.

Prokinetics

Prokinetic agents can theoretically enhance esophageal clearance of refluxed gastric contents by improving peristalsis. The only prokinetic currently available in the United States is metoclopramide, which has been shown to augment LES pressure, increase gastric emptying, and enhance esophageal peristalsis.[48] However, in a randomized double-blind study of patients with EE, metoclopramide failed to improve esophageal acid exposure and esophageal clearance when compared with placebo.[49] In another study, adding metoclopramide to the H2RA ranitidine did not result in any additional benefit for healing EE or controlling reflux symptoms.[50] There are no data to support the use of metoclopramide as an adjunct to PPI therapy. In addition, metoclopramide has important central nervous system side effects including drowsiness, agitation, irritability, depression, and dystonic reactions, and it can cause tardive dyskinesia (the latter in less than 1% of patients).[51] For all of these reasons, metoclopramide is not recommended as a treatment for GERD.[52] Other prokinetics, such as domperidone, itopride, and mosapride, may have modest benefits for the treatment of GERD but studies are limited and none of these agents are available in the United States.[15]

Mucosal repair

Dilation of the intercellular space diameter (ISD) of the esophageal epithelium, measured by transmission electron microscopy, was found to be an early morphologic marker of tissue damage in a GERD animal model.[53] This finding was later confirmed in esophageal biopsies from GERD patients with as well as without EE,[54] and the technique has emerged as a sensitive way to assess esophageal mucosal integrity. A subsequent study found that symptomatic GERD patients have increased ISD; furthermore, treatment with a PPI resulted in normalization of ISD and resolution of heartburn.[55] A more recent study demonstrated that ISD is increased in GERD patients with heartburn that fails to respond to PPI therapy compared with healthy controls.[10] Thus, promoting restoration of esophageal mucosal integrity through other pharmacologic approaches is an attractive idea.

Rebamipide, a cytoprotective antiulcer agent that enhances the production of endogenous prostaglandins, has been recently evaluated for the treatment of GERD. In a study of patients with esophagitis LA classification grade A or B that achieved symptomatic relief after an 8-week course of lansoprazole, maintenance therapy with lansoprazole plus rebamipide resulted in a significantly lower rate of relapse compared with lansoprazole alone.[56] In a more recent study of patients with normal endoscopy who had not achieved symptom relief with a PPI, the addition of rebamipide failed to result in significant improvement when compared with placebo.[57] However, GERD was not confirmed by reflux monitoring so it is possible that some of the patients had a functional GI disorder rather than GERD. Further studies will be needed to clarify the role of rebamipide in GERD.

The serotonin 5-HT$_4$ receptor agonist tegaserod has been shown to have a significant stimulatory impact on several salivary protective factors as well as esophageal epidermal growth factor secretion and may therefore have esophagoprotective properties.[58] In an open-label study of patients that were randomized to tegaserod alone, esomeprazole alone, or tegaserod plus omeprazole, heartburn relief was significantly more frequent with combined therapy compared with either monotherapy.[59] However, tegaserod has been removed from the market because of serious adverse cardiovascular effects.

Modulating Sensation

The final steps in the sequence of events leading to symptoms caused by reflux involves activation of esophageal mucosal nociceptors, firing of afferent signals, and interpretation of these signals in the brain cortex, all of which offer potential therapeutic targets for control of esophageal symptoms.

Nociceptor blockade

Among the several nociceptors that have been identified in the esophagus, the transient receptor potential vanilloid receptor 1 (TRPV1) is regarded as the most important one.[12] TRPV1, a polymodal nonselective calcium-permeable cation channel, is activated by exposure to capsaicin and related natural irritants (referred to as vanilloids), such as heat and acids,[11] and may also play a role in the response to mechanical stimulation such as distension.[60] A recent study demonstrated increased TRPV1 levels in esophageal biopsies from patients with heartburn and erosive as well as nonerosive reflux disease.[61] Therefore, blocking nociceptors could potentially relieve esophageal symptoms.

The TRPV antagonist AZD1386 reduced esophageal pain thresholds in healthy volunteers, but the effect was specific for heat-induced pain and the thresholds for perception of acid infusion or balloon distension were not affected.[62] In a more recent placebo-controlled, double-blind, crossover study that compared AZD1386 to placebo in patients with nonerosive reflux disease and partial PPI response, AZD1386 had no analgesic effect on experimental esophageal pain.[63] Despite these negative results, nociceptor blockade remains an attractive therapeutic target.

Visceral analgesia and cortical modulation

In some patients who do not improve with standard therapies for GERD, there may be a component of visceral hypersensitivity and thus regulating afferent signaling and cortical interpretation of these signals may provide relief. Antidepressant medications may modulate esophageal sensation peripherally at the sensory afferent level, as well as in the central nervous system.[24] In a recent double-blind, randomized, controlled trial the selective serotonin reuptake inhibitor citalopram was compared with placebo in patients with hypersensitive esophagus who complained of typical symptoms (heartburn, regurgitation, chest pain). After 6 months of treatment, ongoing symptoms were significantly less common with citalopram compared with placebo (38% vs 66%).[64] Other treatments that focus on cortical modulation have shown positive effects in small studies. In a controlled trial of guided relaxation compared with a placebo intervention in GERD patients, symptom ratings were significantly lower in the relaxation training group.[65] In patients with heartburn refractory to once-daily PPI who were randomized to acupuncture versus doubling the dose of PPI, acupuncture was found to be superior for symptom control.[66] Other interventions that have been found to be beneficial for functional chest pain may be useful in GERD, including hypnotherapy[67] and Johrei (a therapy based on transmission of healing energy that has been used for chronic pain),[68] but these have not been evaluated specifically in GERD.

SUMMARY

The mainstay of pharmacologic therapy for GERD is gastric acid suppression with PPIs, with generally no major differences among the available PPIs for healing of

EE and achieving symptom control, but definite superiority for these treatment end-points when comparing them with the H2RAs. Despite their proven effectiveness, up to one-third of patients may have insufficient symptomatic relief despite PPI therapy, prompting a search for alternative treatments. The antireflux barrier function can be enhanced with TLESR inhibitors, but at the present time only the GABA-B agonist baclofen is available for this purpose as development of other compounds was stopped because of low efficacy or side effects. Although esophageal defense can be theoretically enhanced by improving esophageal clearance with prokinetics, the efficacy of these agents for this purpose has been limited and side effects are important with metoclopramide, the only currently available prokinetic in the United States. Another avenue for improving esophageal defense is to support the esoph-ageal mucosa with compounds such as rebamipide, which increases endogenous prostaglandin production and has shown a positive impact on maintenance of GERD relief in limited trials. Finally, the sensory pathways responsible for GERD symptoms can be targeted by esophageal mucosal nociceptor blockade or modula-tion of afferent signals and their interpretation in the brain cortex with a variety of compounds or cognitive techniques. Blocking the TRPV1 nociceptor has not resulted in significant improvement of pain thresholds in early studies. Visceral anal-gesia with the selective serotonin reuptake inhibitor citalopram has been shown to be effective for symptom control in patients with hypersensitive esophagus in a ran-domized trial. Cortical modulation with techniques such as relaxation training or acupuncture may also offer benefits to GERD patients, but trials are limited. As can be gleaned from this summary, the data supporting these new and evolving approaches for treating GERD are limited and most of these agents are not ready for routine clinical use. However, further clinical trials and additional insights into the pathophysiology of GERD that can be translated into therapeutic targets are awaited.

REFERENCES

1. Locke GR III, Talley NJ, Fett SL, et al. Prevalence and clinical spectrum of gastroesophageal reflux: a population-based study in Olmsted County, Minne-sota. Gastroenterology 1997;112:1448–56.
2. Peery AF, Dellon ES, Lund J, et al. Burden of gastrointestinal disease in the United States: 2012 update. Gastroenterology 2012;143:1179–87.
3. Gatyas G. IMS Health Reports: US prescription sales in 2009. 2010. Available at: http://www.imshealth.com/portal/site/imshealth/menuitem.a46c6d4df3db4b3d 88f611019418c22a/?vgnextoid=d690a27e9d5b7210VgnVCM100000ed152ca 2RCRD. Accessed October 1, 2013.
4. Fass R, Sifrim D. Management of heartburn not responding to proton pump inhibitors. Gut 2009;58:295–309.
5. Dent J, El-Serag HB, Wallander MA, et al. Epidemiology of gastro-oesophageal disease: a systematic review. Gut 2005;54:710–7.
6. Vela MF. Non-acid reflux: detection, clinical significance and management. The role of multichannel intraluminal impedance (MII-pH) testing. Am J Gastroen-terol 2009;104:277–80.
7. Barlow WJ, Orlando RC. The pathogenesis of heartburn in nonerosive reflux dis-ease: a unifying hypothesis. Gastroenterology 2005;128:771–8.
8. Weijenborg PW, Kessing BF, Smout AJ. Gastroesophageal reflux disease: path-ophysiology. In: Vela MF, Pandolfino JE, Richter JE, editors. Practical manual of GERD. Oxford (UK): Wiley; 2013. p. 3–25.

9. Tutuian R, Vela MF, Hill E, et al. Characteristics of symptomatic reflux episodes on acid suppressive therapy. Am J Gastroenterol 2008;103:1090–6.

10. Vela MF, Craft BM, Sharma N, et al. Refractory heartburn: comparison of intercellular space diameter in documented GERD vs. functional heartburn. Am J Gastroenterol 2011;106:844–50.

11. Sieh KR, Yi CH, Liu TT, et al. Evidence for neurotrophic factors associating with TRPV1 gene expression in the inflamed human esophagus. Neurogastroenterol Motil 2010;22:971–8.

12. Banerjee B, Medda BK, Lazarova Z, et al. Effect of reflux-induced inflammation on transient receptor potential vanilloid one (TRPV1) expression in primary sensory neurons innervating the oesophagus of rats. Neurogastroenterol Motil 2007;19:681–91.

13. Miwa H, Kondo T, Oshima T, et al. Esophageal sensation and esophageal hypersensitivity – overview from bench to bedside. J Neurogastroenterol Motil 2010; 16:353–62.

14. Katz PO, Stein EM. Medical management of gastroesophageal reflux disease. In: Richter JE, Castell DO, editors. The esophagus. Oxford (UK): Wiley; 2012.

15. Hershcovici T, Fass R. Gastro-oesophageal reflux disease. Beyond proton pump inhibitor therapy. Drugs 2011;71:2381–9.

16. Chiba N, De Gara CJ, Wilkinson JM, et al. Speed of healing and symptom relief in grade II to IV gastroesophageal reflux disease: a meta-analysis. Gastroenterology 1997;112:1798–810.

17. Peghini PL, Katz PO, Castell DO. Ranitidine controls nocturnal gastric acid breakthrough on omeprazole: a control study in normal subjects. Gastroenterology 1998;115:1335–9.

18. Fackler WK, Ours TM, Vaezi MF, et al. Long-term effect of H2RA therapy on nocturnal gastric acid breakthrough. Gastroenterology 2002;122:625–32.

19. Gralnek IM, Dulai GS, Fennerty MB, et al. Esomeprazole versus other proton pump inhibitors in erosive esophagitis: a meta-analysis of randomized clinical trials. Clin Gastroenterol Hepatol 2006;4:1452–8.

20. Castell DO, Bagin R, Goldlust B, et al. Comparison of the effects of immediate-release omeprazole powder for oral suspension and pantoprazole delayed-release tablets on nocturnal acid breakthrough in patients with symptomatic gastro-oesophageal reflux disease. Aliment Pharmacol Ther 2005;21:1467–74.

21. Sharma P, Shaheen NJ, Perez MC, et al. Clinical trials: healing of erosive esophagitis with dexlansoprazole MR, a proton pump inhibitor with a novel dual delayed-release formulation – results from two randomized controlled studies. Aliment Pharmacol Ther 2009;29:731–41.

22. Fass R, Sontag SJ, Traxler B, et al. Treatment of patients with persistent heartburn symptoms: a double-blind, randomized trial. Clin Gastroenterol Hepatol 2006;4:50–6.

23. Fass R, Murthy U, Hayden CW, et al. Omeprazole 40 mg once a day is equally effective as lansoprazole 30 mg twice a day in symptom control of patients with gastroesophageal reflux disease who are resistant to conventional-dose lansoprazole therapy – a prospective, randomized, multi-centre study. Aliment Pharmacol Ther 2000;14:1595–603.

24. Roman S, Kharilas PJ. Overview of GERD treatments. In: Vela MF, Pandolfino JE, Richter JE, editors. Practical manual of GERD. Oxford (UK): Wiley; 2013. p. 53–68.

25. Galmiche JP, Hatlebakk J, Attwood S, et al. Laparoscopic antireflux surgery vs esomeprazole treatment for chronic GERD. The LOTUS randomized clinical trial. JAMA 2011;305:1969–77.

26. Scarpignato C, Hunt RH. Proton pump inhibitors: the beginning of the end or the end of the beginning? Curr Opin Pharmacol 2008;8:677–84.

27. Kharilas PJ, Dent J, Lauritsen K, et al. A randomized, comparative study of three doses of AZD8065 and esomeprazole for healing of reflux esophagitis. Clin Gastroenterol Hepatol 2007;5:1385–91.

28. Vela MF, Camacho-Lobato L, Srinivasan R, et al. Intraesophageal impedance and pH measurement of acid and non-acid reflux: effect of omeprazole. Gastroenterology 2001;120:1599–606.

29. Zerbib F, Roman S, Ropert A, et al. Esophageal pH-impedance monitoring and symptom analysis in GERD: a study in patients off and on therapy. Am J Gastroenterol 2006;101:1956–63.

30. Boeckxstaens GE, Smout A. Systematic review: role of acid, weakly acidic and weakly alkaline reflux in gastro-oesophageal reflux disease. Aliment Pharmacol Ther 2010;32:334–43.

31. Frazzoni M, Conigliaro R, Melotti G. Reflux parameters as modified by laparoscopic fundoplication in 40 patients with heartburn/regurgitation persisting despite PPI therapy: a study using impedance-pH monitoring. Dig Dis Sci 2011;56:1099–106.

32. Mittal RK, Holloway RH, Penagini R, et al. Transient lower esophageal sphincter relaxation. Gastroenterology 1995;109:601–10.

33. Kessing BF, Conchillo JM, Bredenoord AJ, et al. Review article: the clinical relevance of transient lower esophageal sphincter relaxations in gastro-oesophageal reflux disease. Aliment Pharmacol Ther 2011;33:650–61.

34. Dent J. Reflux inhibitor drugs: an emerging novel therapy for gastroesophageal reflux disease. J Dig Dis 2010;11:72–5.

35. Zhang Q, Lehmann A, Ridga R, et al. Control of transient lower oesophageal sphincter relaxations and reflux by the GABA(B) agonist baclofen in patients with gastroesophageal reflux disease. Gut 2002;50:19–24.

36. Vela MF, Tutuian R, Katz PO, et al. Baclofen decreases acid and non-acid postprandial gastro-oesophageal reflux measured by combined multichannel intraluminal impedance and pH. Aliment Pharmacol Ther 2003;17:243–51.

37. Orr WC, Goodrich S, Wright S, et al. The effect of baclofen on nocturnal gastroesophageal reflux and measures of sleep quality: a randomized, cross-over trial. Neurogastroenterol Motil 2012;24:553–9.

38. Koek GH, Sifrim D, Lerut T, et al. Effect of the GABA(B) agonist baclofen in patients with symptoms and duodeno-gastro-oesophageal reflux refractory to proton pump inhibitors. Gut 2003;52:1397–402.

39. Boeckxstaens GE, Rydholm H, Lei A, et al. Effect of lesogaberan, a novel GABA(B)-receptor agonist, on transient lower oesophageal sphincter relaxations in male subjects. Aliment Pharmacol Ther 2010;31:1208–17.

40. Boeckxstaens GE, Beaumont H, Hatlebakk JG, et al. A novel reflux inhibitor lesogaberan (AZD3355) as add-on treatment in patients with GORD with persistent reflux symptoms despite proton pump inhibitor therapy: a randomized placebo-controlled trial. Gut 2011;60:1182–8.

41. Gerson LB, Huff FJ, Hila A, et al. Arbaclofen placarbil decreases postprandial reflux in patients with gastroesophageal reflux disease. Am J Gastroenterol 2010;105:1266–75.

42. Vakil NB, Huff FJ, Bian A, et al. Arbaclofen placarbil in GERD: a randomized, double-blind, placebo-controlled study. Am J Gastroenterol 2011;106:1427–38.

43. Keywood C, Wakefiled M, Tack J. A proof-of-concept study evaluating the effect of ADX10059, a metabotropic glutamate receptor-5 negative allosteric

modulator, on acid exposure and symptoms in gastro-oesophageal reflux disease. Gut 2009;58:1192–9.

44. Rohof WO, Lei A, Hirsch DP, et al. The effects of a novel metabotropic glutamate receptor-5 antagonist AZD2066 on transient lower oesophageal sphincter relaxations. Aliment Pharmacol Ther 2012;35:1231–42.

45. Beaumont H, Jensen J, Carlsson A, et al. Effect of delta9-tetrahydrocannabinol, a cannabinoid receptor agonist, on the triggering of transient lower oesophageal sphincter relaxations in dogs and humans. Br J Pharmacol 2009;156:153–62.

46. Scarpellini E, Blondeau K, Boeckxstaens V, et al. Effect of rimonabant on esophageal motor function in man. Aliment Pharmacol Ther 2011;33:730–7.

47. Trudgill NJ, Hussain FN, Moustafa M, et al. The effect of cholecystokinin antagonism on postprandial lower oesophageal sphincter function an asymptomatic volunteers and patients with reflux disease. Aliment Pharmacol Ther 2001;15:1357–64.

48. Champion MC. Prokinetic therapy in gastroesophageal reflux disease. Can J Gastroenterol 1997;11(Suppl B):55B–65B.

49. Grande L, Lacima G, Ros E, et al. Lack of effect of metoclopramide and domperidone on esophageal peristalsis and esophageal acid clearance in reflux esophagitis. A randomized, double-blind study. Dig Dis Sci 1992;37:583–8.

50. Richter JE, Sabesin SM, Kogut DG, et al. Omperazole versus ranitidine or ranitidine/metoclopramide in poorly responsive symptomatic gastroesophageal reflux disease. Am J Gastroenterol 1996;91:1766–72.

51. Rao AS, Camilleri M. Review article: metoclopramide and tardive dyskinesia. Aliment Pharmacol Ther 2010;31:11–9.

52. Katz PO, Gerson LB, Vela MF. Guidelines for the diagnosis and management of gastroesophageal reflux disease. Am J Gastroenterol 2013;108:308–28.

53. Orlando RC, Powell DW, Carney CN. Pathophysiology of acute acid injury in rabbit esophageal epithelium. J Clin Invest 1981;68:286–93.

54. Tobey NA, Carson JL, Alkiek RA, et al. Dilated intercellular spaces: a morphological feature of acid reflux–damaged human esophageal epithelium. Gastroenterology 1996;111:1200–5.

55. Calabrese C, Bortolotti M, Fabbri A, et al. Reversibility of GERD Ultrastructural alterations and relief of symptoms after omeprazole treatment. Am J Gastroenterol 2005;100:537–42.

56. Yoshida N, Kamada K, Tomatsuri N, et al. Management of recurrence of symptoms of gastroesophageal reflux disease: synergistic effect of rebamipide with 15mg lansoprazole. Dig Dis Sci 2010;55:3393–8.

57. Adachi K, Furuta K, Miwa H, et al. A study on the efficacy of rebamipide for patients with proton pump inhibitor-refractory non-erosive reflux disease. Dig Dis Sci 2012;57:1609–17.

58. Majewski M, Jaworski T, Sarosiek I, et al. Significant enhancement of esophageal pre-epithelial defense by tegaserod: implications for an esophagoprotective effect. Clin Gastroenterol Hepatol 2007;5:430–8.

59. Zeng J, Zuo XL, Li YQ, et al. Tegaserod for dyspepsia and reflux symptoms in patients with chronic constipation: an exploratory open-label study. Eur J Clin Pharmacol 2007;63:529–36.

60. Blelefeldt K, Davis BM. Differential effects of ASIC3 and TRPV1 deletion on gastroesophageal sensation in mice. Am J Physiol Gastrointest Liver Physiol 2008;294:G130–8.

61. Guarino MP, Cheng L, Ma J, et al. Increased TRPV1 gene expression in esophageal mucosa of patients with non-erosive and erosive reflux disease. Neurogastroenterol Motil 2010;22:746–52.

62. Krarup AL, Ny L, Astrand M, et al. Randomised clinical trial: the efficacy of a transient receptor potential vanilloid 1 antagonist AZD1386 in human oesophageal pain. Aliment Pharmacol Ther 2011;33:1113–22.

63. Krarup AL, Ny L, Gunnarsson J, et al. Randomised clinical trial: inhibition of the TRPV1 system in patients with nonerosive gastroesophageal reflux disease and a partial response to PPI treatment is not associated with analgesia to esophageal experimental pain. Scand J Gastroenterol 2013;48:274–84.

64. Viazis N, Keyoglou A, Kanellopoulos AK, et al. Selective serotonin reuptake inhibitors for the treatment of hypersensitive esophagus: a randomized, double-blind, placebo controlled study. Am J Gastroenterol 2012;107:1662–7.

65. McDonald-Haile J, Braley LA, Bailey MA, et al. Relaxation training reduces symptom reports and acid exposure in patients with gastroesophageal reflux disease. Gastroenterology 1994;107:61–9.

66. Dickman R, Schiff E, Holland A, et al. Clinical trial: acupuncture vs. doubling the proton pump inhibitor dose in refractory heartburn. Aliment Pharmacol Ther 2007;26:1333–44.

67. Jones H, Cooper P, Miller V, et al. Treatment of non-cardiac chest pain: a controlled trial of hypnotherapy. Gut 2006;55:1403–8.

68. Gasiorowska A, Navarro-Rodriguez T, Dickman R, et al. Clinical trial: the effect of Johrei on symptoms of patients with functional chest pain. Aliment Pharmacol Ther 2008;29:126–34.

Surgical Treatment of GERD
Where Have We Been and Where Are We Going?

David Kim, MD, Vic Velanovich, MD*

KEYWORDS

- Gastroesophageal reflux disease • Open antireflux surgery
- Laparoscopic antireflux surgery • Endoscopic antireflux surgery

KEY POINTS

- Surgical management of gastroesophageal reflux disease has evolved from relatively invasive procedures requiring open laparotomy or thoracotomy to minimally invasive laparoscopic techniques.
- Although side effects may still occur after gastroesophageal reflux disease operations, with careful patient selection and good technique, the overall symptomatic control leads to satisfaction rates in the 90% range.
- Newer laparoscopically placed devices hold promise in achieving equivalent symptomatic relief with fewer side effects.

HISTORICAL REVIEW

Philip Allison first emphasized the association between reflux esophagitis and hiatal hernia in 1951.[1] This lead surgeons to explore surgical options in the management of gastroesophageal reflux disease (GERD) and hiatal hernia. Although it is now clear that lower esophageal sphincter (LES) competence is a multifactorial system, initial operations focused on hiatal hernia repair.

Allison first attempted simple reduction of the herniated stomach with repair of the hiatal hernia.[1] Results, however, were unsatisfactory. The next iteration incorporated augmentation of the LES. It was first described by Rudolph Nissen in 1956.[2] Originally, the anterior and posterior walls of the fundus were used for the fundoplication without division of the short gastric vessels; this was wrapped around 6 cm of distal esophagus just above the gastroesophageal junction and approximated using 4 or 5 interrupted sutures, of which one or more incorporated the anterior wall of the

Division of General Surgery, University of South Florida, One Tampa General Circle, Tampa, FL 33606, USA
* Corresponding author. Division of General Surgery, University of South Florida, One Tampa General Circle, F145, Tampa, FL 33606.
E-mail address: vvelanov@health.usf.edu

Gastroenterol Clin N Am 43 (2014) 135–145
http://dx.doi.org/10.1016/j.gtc.2013.12.002   gastro.theclinics.com
0889-8553/14/$ – see front matter © 2014 Elsevier Inc. All rights reserved.

esophagus. The fundoplication was performed over a 36-Fr esophageal bougie dilator. Of note, Nissen did not repair the crura in his original description.

The original Nissen fundoplication had relatively unacceptable postoperative incidences of dysphagia and gas-bloat. It was thought that the fundoplication was "too long and too tight." In an effort to minimize these, modifications were made to the original Nissen fundoplication without decreasing its effectiveness in preventing pathologic reflux. Donahue and coworkers described using a larger 50-Fr esophageal bougie during the creation of the fundoplication in association with hiatal hernia repair.[3] Following this, DeMeester and his group[4] described several other measures that improved the postoperative outcome of fundoplication. These measures included using a larger 60-Fr esophageal bougie, decreasing the length of the gastric wrap to 1 cm, and dividing the short gastric vessels to use the gastric fundus in constructing a "floppy" wrap. The final step was to insert an index finger along the esophagus while the 60-Fr bougie was in place to ensure that the wrap was sufficiently "floppy" (**Fig. 1**).[4] The Nissen fundoplication enhances LES competence by placing the distal 2 cm of the esophagus in the intra-abdominal position, restoring the interaction of the distal esophagus with the diaphragmatic hiatus, and augmenting the distal esophageal musculature with the fundoplication. Although much is made of the fundoplication, it consists of all 3 components working in concert, allowing for correction of pathologic reflux and symptomatic improvement. Rossetti and Hell modified the Nissen by using only the anterior wall of the gastric fundus.[5] Despite these modifications and success in eliminating reflux, the Nissen fundoplication has been associated with side effects of bloating, dysphagia, and diarrhea.[6]

Other surgical options have been described but are not nearly as popular as the modified Nissen fundoplication. André Toupet[7] in 1963 described a posterior 270° wrap as an alternative to the Nissen fundoplication to decrease the incidence of postoperative bloating and dysphagia (**Fig. 2**). The results vary in comparison with the Nissen fundoplication. Certainly, although dysphagia is less compared with the Nissen, long-term durability is a problem.[8] Currently, the Toupet posterior fundoplication is generally reserved for patients with abnormal esophageal motility with similar results to the Nissen fundoplication,[9] although there are some groups that advocate its routine use. Dor[10] created a 180° anterior fundoplication used primarily in combination with Heller esophagomyotomy for achalasia; it can be used as a primary surgical treatment for GERD. Recent data do not show a difference in outcome between the anterior partial fundoplication and the posterior partial fundoplication.

For patients with severe esophagitis leading to stricturing, there was concern that recurrent hiatal hernia could occur because of esophageal foreshortening. Because of this, Collis created an "esophageal lengthening" procedure to insure an intra-abdominal esophagus, consisting of placing a dilator in the esophagus and gastric cardia, then dividing the gastric cardia from the angle of His parallel to the dilator for a distance of 2 to 3 cm. The fundoplication was then completed around this "neo-esophagus" and the hiatal defect was repaired. In the 1960s, Belsy described an imbricating partial fundoplication completed in the left thoracic cavity (**Fig. 3**). These operations all required a laparotomy or left thoracotomy for completion.

For decades, these operations have been the mainstay of surgical treatment of hiatal hernia and GERD. However, their application was relatively uncommon compared with the prevalence disease despite evidence of their superiority to medical management of reflux,[7,8] attributed primarily to concern over side effects and the relatively invasive nature of these surgical treatments.

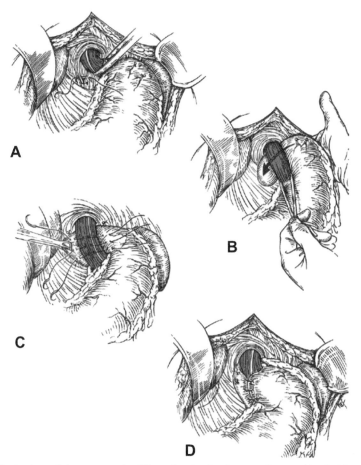

Fig. 1. Illustration of the present-day Nissen fundoplication as advocated by DeMeester. Key components include reduction of the herniated stomach with at least 2 cm of intra-abdominal esophagus, repair of the hiatal hernia defect posterior to the esophagus, division of the short gastric vessels to allow for both mobilization of the and view of the posterior surface of the fundus, and a 360° fundoplication over a large-bore dilator. (*From* Ferguson MK. Atlas of esophageal surgery. In: Bell RH Jr, Rikkers LF, Mulholland MW, editors. Digestive tract surgery: a text and atlas. Philadelphia: Lippincott-Raven Publishers; 1996. p. 107–63; with permission.)

DEVELOPMENT OF LAPAROSCOPIC ANTIREFLUX SURGERY

With the advent of laparoscopic cholecystectomy in the late 1980s, surgeons began to explore other operations that could be done laparoscopically. In 1991 Dallemagne and coworkers first reported the feasibility of laparoscopic Nissen fundoplication.[11] As laparoscopic antireflux surgery entered into practice, the number of antireflux operations began to increase, eventually peaking in the United States in 2000 at 32,980 procedures from 9173 procedures in 1993,[12] probably due to patients and referring physicians being more willing to undergo and refer patients for a more "minimally invasive" approach. This trend reversed with the rates of antireflux surgery decreasing by

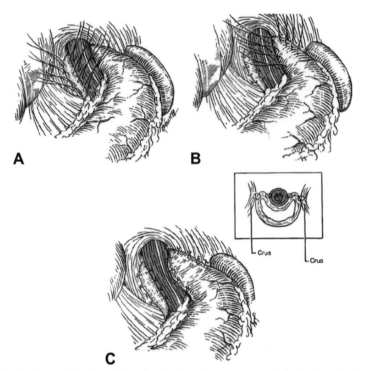

Fig. 2. Illustration of the Toupet fundoplication. Key components include reduction of the herniated stomach and a posterior fundoplication securing the fundus to the right and left crura and to the right and left of the esophagus, leaving a gap of about 120°. Initially, the crural defect was not repaired, but many surgeons now think hiatal repair is important. (*From* Ferguson MK. Atlas of esophageal surgery. In: Bell RH Jr, Rikkers LF, Mulholland MW, editors. Digestive tract surgery: a text and atlas. Philadelphia: Lippincott-Raven Publishers; 1996. p. 107–63; with permission.)

40% by 2006 to 19,668 procedures.[12] Some reasons for this include widespread use of proton pump inhibitor medications (PPIs), patient and physician fear of operation-related side effects, and perioperative complications.

With the resurgence of antireflux surgery in the 1990s, the number of failed antireflux operations also increased. Failures can be categorized as physiologic or anatomic. Physiologic failures are generally due to poor patient selection or adverse alternations in gastrointestinal function. Anatomic failures are related to disruption or poor construction of the fundoplication, a "slipped" fundoplication, a herniated fundoplication, or recurrent hiatal hernia, either a sliding type or a paraesophageal type.[13]

Naturally this led to increased rates of redo fundoplications. Reoperative antireflux surgery is not as effective as a primary procedure; however, upwards of 90% of patients will have good outcomes and most redo procedures can be completed laparoscopically.[14] In 2005, Smith and colleagues[15] reported a low 2.8% failure rate requiring reoperation of 1892 patients undergoing antireflux surgery over 13 years. Most were early failures; 73% required reoperation within the first 2 years of the original surgery, and the most common mechanism of failure was transdiaphragmatic wrap herniation (61%).

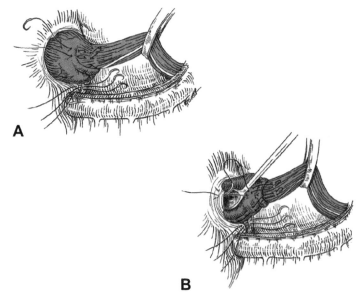

Fig. 3. Illustration of a Belsey fundoplication. This operation required a thoracotomy. The key components were bringing the stomach into the posterior mediastinum and suturing in 2 layers for 270° around the esophagus. (*From* Ferguson MK. Atlas of esophageal surgery. In: Bell RH Jr, Rikkers LF, Mulholland MW, editors. Digestive tract surgery: a text and atlas. Philadelphia: Lippincott-Raven Publishers; 1996. p. 107–63; with permission.)

KEYS IN PATIENT SELECTION

Antireflux surgery is very successful in appropriately selected patients. The preoperative evaluation should include documentation of increased esophageal acid exposure with ambulatory 24- or 48-hour pH monitoring, assessment of esophageal motility using esophageal manometry, and upper gastrointestinal endoscopy in every patient.[16] Preoperative assessment of esophageal motility is important to help elucidate any underlying motility disorder that may be the cause of a patient's symptoms and preclude fundoplication. Upper endoscopy provides objective evidence of mucosal damage, presence of Barrett's metaplasia or esophageal neoplasia, and size of an associated hiatal hernia.

Indications for laparoscopic antireflux surgery[17]:

- Complications of GERD unresponsive to medical therapy with associated GERD-related symptoms
  - Esophagitis
  - Stricture
  - Recurrent aspiration or pneumonia
  - Barrett esophagus
- Continued symptoms despite maximal medical treatment
- Symptomatic paraesophageal hernia
- Patient desire to discontinue PPI therapy
  - Financial burden
  - Lifestyle choice
  - Young age
- Intolerance or adverse events related to acid suppressive medications

Indications for partial fundoplication[17]:

- Poor esophageal clearance because of esophageal motility abnormality
- Severe aerophagia, particularly in patients with daytime reflux associated with belching
- Insufficient gastric fundus to allow a loose total fundoplication
- Psychological inability to tolerate the side effects of fundoplication
- In association with Heller myotomy for achalasia

PREDICTORS OF SUCCESS

As previously mentioned, laparoscopic antireflux surgery controls symptoms of GERD reliably in well-selected patients. There are several aspects of the preoperative evaluation that predict success. Abnormal 24-hour pH scores are the strongest predictor of success (odds ratio = 5.1; 95% CI = 1.9–15.3),[18] followed by typical primary symptoms of GERD (odds ratio = 5.1; 95% CI = 1.9–13.6) and a clinical response to acid suppression therapy (odds ratio = 3.3; 95% CI = 1.3–8.7).[18] Typical symptoms of GERD are heartburn, regurgitation, and dysphagia. The combination of typical symptoms responding to acid-suppressing medication with abnormal pH monitoring while off of these medications will lead to symptomatic improvement in more than 90% of patients after antireflux operations. Other symptoms of GERD that are considered atypical include hoarseness, cough, wheezing, and chest pain. In patients whose primary symptoms of GERD are atypical, the success of antireflux surgery is far less.

Conversely, several factors have been identified as predictive of failure after laparoscopic antireflux surgery. These factors include large hiatal hernia, which leads to symptomatic failure and not necessarily a higher rate of recurrent hiatal hernia and failure to respond to PPI therapy preoperatively, predominately upright, daytime reflux, severe esophageal dysmotility disorders, such as scleroderma or ineffective esophageal motility, and the presence of functional gastrointestinal disorders.[19,20] Interestingly, a history of psycho-emotional disorders and chronic pain problems is also associated with poor GERD-related symptom control and other adverse symptomatic events after antireflux surgery for GERD.[21–23]

KEYS IN OPERATIVE TECHNIQUE

The goals of laparoscopic antireflux surgery are to restore an effective LES. DeMeester's group[24] described a standardized approach to antireflux surgery to attempt to improve outcomes by adhering to 10 technical principles of a Nissen fundoplication

- Right vagus identified
- Left vagus identified
- Hepatic branch of vagus preserved
- Cardioesophageal fat pad removed
- Gastric fundus mobilized by division of short gastrics
- Closure of crura
- Wrap placed between right vagus and esophagus
- Teflon pledgets used
- Bougie used to quantitate wrap size
- Length of wrap ≤2 cm

Adherence to the previous 10 techniques has been shown to

1. Restore the overall manometric length of the distal esophageal sphincter to at least 3 cm and its pressure to a level 2 times resting gastric pressure
2. Place an adequate length of the distal esophageal sphincter in the positive pressure environment of the abdomen
3. Ensure that the reconstructed cardia relaxes on deglutition and does not increase the outflow resistance of the relaxed sphincter to a level that exceeds the peristaltic power of the body of the esophagus
4. Ensure that the fundoplication remains within the abdomen

These steps led to a relief of symptoms in 93% of patients and a 77% rate of healing of esophagitis.[24]

In 1999, Bowerey and Peters[25] reiterated many of these steps to maximize success of a laparoscopic Nissen fundoplication. They stressed the importance of crural closure, complete mobilization of the fundus by dividing the short gastrics, and creating a short, loose fundoplication composed of the anterior and posterior fundic walls around the esophagus.

ENDOSCOPIC ANTIREFLUX SURGERY

The success of minimally invasive antireflux surgery has spurred interest in even more minimally invasive approaches to GERD treatment, leading to several endoscopic and/or endoluminal treatments for GERD. The EndoCinch device leads to the development of the endoluminal gastroplication procedure, aimed to augment the LES by forming pleats in the sphincter using stitches (**Fig. 4**). This procedure had poor long-term results and is no longer available on the market.[26] Another endoluminal technique that is no longer available was the NDO Surgical Plicator by NDO Surgical Inc (Mansfield, MA, USA). This device aimed to plicate tissue near the gastroesophageal junction, fixing it using a suture-based implant. However, the company ceased operations in 2008.

The 2 currently available endoluminal treatments for GERD were reviewed by the Society of American Gastrointestinal and Endoscopic Surgeons (SAGES) in 2013. The EsophyX device by Endogastric Solutions (Redwood City, WA, USA) was designed to perform transoral incisionless fundoplication and was first approved by

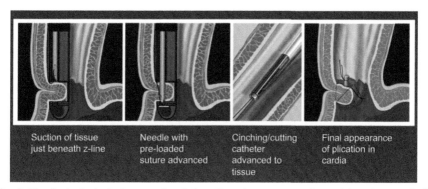

| Suction of tissue just beneath z-line | Needle with pre-loaded suture advanced | Cinching/cutting catheter advanced to tissue | Final appearance of plication in cardia |

Fig. 4. The Endocinch device creating "pleats" at the gastroesophageal junction to "bulk up" the lower esophageal sphincter. (*Courtesy of* Bard Medical, Covington, GA; with permission. Copyright © 2013 CR Bard Inc.)

the Food and Drug Administration in 2007 (**Fig. 5**). It uses "H-shaped" fasteners made of polypropylene to create a full-thickness plication. After reviewing the available literature SAGES concluded that in the short term (6 months to 2 years) the EsophyX device may be effective in patients with hiatal hernia less than 2 cm, with typical and atypical symptoms of GERD, although long-term data are not available.[27] The Stretta system by Mederi Therapeutics Inc (Greenwich, CT, USA) was approved for use by the Food and Drug Administration in 2000 (**Fig. 6**). Using radiofrequency, the Stretta system remodels the musculature of the LES and gastric cardia, reducing tissue compliance and transient LES relaxations, which restore the natural barrier function of the LES and decreases regurgitation. On review of the literature SAGES gave a strong recommendation to the use of Stretta for patients 18 years or older with symptoms of GERD for more than 6 months who do not desire laparoscopic fundoplication.[27]

The main issues involved with endoluminal treatments of GERD have been durability of symptomatic relief and actual correction of pathologic reflux. Although initial symptomatic improvement was good in most devices, long-term remission of

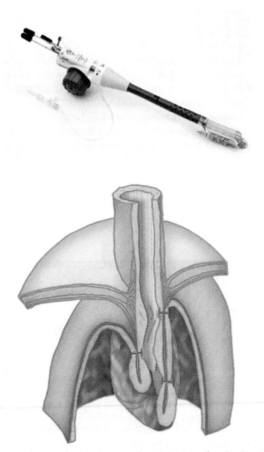

Fig. 5. The Esophyx device and the transoral incisionless fundoplication. (*Courtesy of* Endogastric Solutions, San Mateo, CA; with permission. © 2013 EndoGastric Solutions, Inc.)

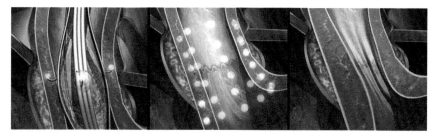

Fig. 6. The Stretta system for application of radiofrequency energy to the gastroesophageal junction. (*Courtesy of* Mederi Therapeutics, Greenwich, CT; with permission. © 2013 Mederi Therapeutics Inc.)

GERD-related symptoms was low. Therefore, many third-party payors have placed a moratorium on payment for any endoluminal antireflux procedure. Although some insurance companies will reimburse for these procedures, many will not.

FUTURE DEVELOPMENTS

There are several newer products currently under evaluation that show some promising initial results. The LINX reflux management system by Torax Medical, Inc (Shoreview, MN, USA) augments the LES using a series of magnetic beads that are connected by titanium links (**Fig. 7**). This configuration allows the system to open during swallowing or belching. Initial data have demonstrated symptomatic improvement, although not complete elimination of pathologic reflux. The side-effect profile appears better than with traditional Nissen fundoplication.[28] Comparative trials and long-term data are necessary to determine the place of this procedure in the treatment of GERD.[29] Nevertheless, the initial results are promising. The SAGES Technology Assessment and Value Analysis task force has concluded that the Linx device is safe and effective for the management of GERD (www.sages.org, lasted accessed October 1, 2013).[30] Last, the EndoStim LES Stimulation System by EndoStim BV (The Hague, Netherlands) aims to increase LES pressure without interfering with LES relaxation by using temporary electrical stimulation of the LES. This system requires a permanently implanted stimulator. Early results are promising but long-term data are lacking.[31] The device is entering into clinical trials.

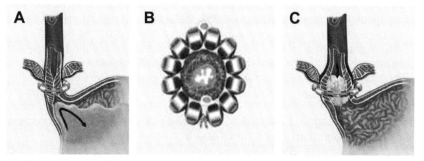

Fig. 7. The Linx system for the augmentation of the lower esophageal sphincter. (*Courtesy of* Torax Medical, Inc, St Paul, MN; with permission. © 2013 Torax Medical Inc.)

SUMMARY

Surgical management of GERD has evolved from relatively invasive procedures requiring open laparotomy or thoracotomy to minimally invasive laparoscopic techniques. The operation itself has evolved from a fundoplication that was "too long and too tight" associated with a disturbingly high incidence of bloating and dysphagia to one that is "short and floppy." Although side effects may still occur, with careful patient selection and good technique, the overall symptomatic control leads to satisfaction rates in the 90% range. Unfortunately, the next evolution to endoluminal techniques has not been as successful. Reliable devices are still awaited that consistently produce long-term symptomatic relief with correction of pathologic reflux. However, newer laparoscopically placed devices may hold promise in achieving equivalent symptomatic relief with event fewer side effects. Clinical trials are still forthcoming.

REFERENCES

1. Allison PR. Reflux esophagitis, sliding hiatal hernia, and the anatomy of repair. Surg Gynecol Obstet 1951;92(4):419–31.
2. Nissen R. A simple operation for control of reflux esophagitis. Schweiz Med Wochenschr 1956;86(Suppl 20):590–2 [in German].
3. Donahue PE, Samelson S, Nyhus LM, et al. The floppy Nissen fundoplication. Effective long-term control of pathologic reflux. Arch Surg 1985;120(6):663–8.
4. DeMeester TR, Bonavina L, Albertucci M. Nissen fundoplication for gastroesophageal reflux disease. Evaluation of primary repair in 100 consecutive patients. Ann Surg 1986;204(1):9–20.
5. Rossetti M, Hell K. Fundoplication for the treatment of gastroesophageal reflux in hiatal hernia. World J Surg 1977;1(4):439–43.
6. Spechler SJ. Comparison of medical and surgical therapy for complicated gastroesophageal reflux disease in veterans. The Department of Veterans Affairs Gastroesophageal Reflux Disease Study Group. N Engl J Med 1992;326(12):786–92.
7. Toupet A. Technic of esophago-gastroplasty with phrenogastropexy used in radical treatment of hiatal hernias as a supplement to Heller's operation in cardiospasms. Mem Acad Chir (Paris) 1963;89:384–9 [in French].
8. Horvath KD, Jobe BA, Herron DM, et al. Laparoscopic toupet fundoplication is an inadequate procedure for patients with severe reflux disease. J Gastrointest Surg 1999;3(6):583–91.
9. Wetscher GJ, Glaser K, Wieschemeyer T, et al. Tailored antireflux surgery for gastroesophageal reflux disease: effectiveness and risk of postoperative dysphagia. World J Surg 1997;21(6):605–10.
10. Rawlings A, Soper N, Oelschlager B, et al. Laparoscopic Dor versus Toupet fundoplication following Heller myotomy for achalasia: results of a multicenter, prospective, randomized-controlled trial. Surg Endosc 2012;26(1):18–26.
11. Dallemagne B, Weerts JM, Jehaes C, et al. Laparoscopic Nissen fundoplication: preliminary report. Surg Laparosc Endosc 1991;1(3):138–43.
12. Wang YR, Dempsey DT, Richter JE. Trends and perioperative outcomes of inpatient antireflux surgery in the United States, 1993-2006. Dis Esophagus 2011; 24(4):215–23.
13. Soper NJ, Dunnegan D. Anatomic fundoplication failure after laparoscopic antireflux surgery. Ann Surg 1999;229(5):669–76 [discussion: 676–7].
14. Byrne JP, Smithers BM, Nathanson LK, et al. Symptomatic and functional outcome after laparoscopic reoperation for failed antireflux surgery. Br J Surg 2005;92(8):996–1001.

15. Smith CD, McClusky DA, Rajad MA, et al. When fundoplication fails: redo? Ann Surg 2005;241(6):861–9 [discussion: 869–71].
16. Niebisch S, Peters JH. Update on fundoplication for the treatment of GERD. Curr Gastroenterol Rep 2012;14(3):189–96.
17. Fischer JE. Fischer's mastery of surgery. 6th edition. Philadelphia: Wolters Kluwer Health/Lippincott Williams & Wilkins; 2012.
18. Campos GM, Peters JH, DeMeester TR, et al. Multivariate analysis of factors predicting outcome after laparoscopic Nissen fundoplication. J Gastrointest Surg 1999;3(3):292–300.
19. Power C, Maguire D, McAnena O. Factors contributing to failure of laparoscopic Nissen fundoplication and the predictive value of preoperative assessment. Am J Surg 2004;187(4):457–63.
20. Stein HJ, Feussner H, Siewert JR. Failure of antireflux surgery: causes and management strategies. Am J Surg 1996;171(1):36–9 [discussion: 39–40].
21. Kamolz T, Velanovich V. Psychological and emotional aspects of gastroesophageal reflux disease. Dis Esophagus 2002;15(3):199–203.
22. Velanovich V, Karmy-Jones R. Psychiatric disorders affect outcomes of antireflux operations for gastroesophageal reflux disease. Surg Endosc 2001;15(2):171–5.
23. Velanovich V. Nonsurgical factors affecting symptomatic outcomes of antireflux surgery. Dis Esophagus 2006;19(1):1–4.
24. Dunnington GL, DeMeester TR. Outcome effect of adherence to operative principles of Nissen fundoplication by multiple surgeons. The Department of Veterans Affairs Gastroesophageal Reflux Disease Study Group. Am J Surg 1993;166(6):654–7 [discussion: 657–9].
25. Bowrey DJ, Peters JH. Current state, techniques, and results of laparoscopic antireflux surgery. Semin Laparosc Surg 1999;6(4):194–212.
26. Jafri SM, Arora G, Triadafilopoulos G. What is left of the endoscopic antireflux devices? Curr Opin Gastroenterol 2009;25(4):352–7.
27. Auyang ED, Carter P, Rauth T, et al. SAGES clinical spotlight review: endoluminal treatments for gastroesophageal reflux disease (GERD). Surg Endosc 2013;27(8):2658–72.
28. Ganz RA, Peters JH, Horgan S. Esophageal sphincter device for gastroesophageal reflux disease. N Engl J Med 2013;368(21):2039–40.
29. Bonavina L, Saino G, Lipgam JC, et al. LINX((R)) Reflux Management System in chronic gastroesophageal reflux: a novel effective technology for restoring the natural barrier to reflux. Therap Adv Gastroenterol 2013;6(4):261–8.
30. Gould J, Oleynikov D, Rattner D, et al. TAVAc safety and effectiveness analysis: Linx reflux management system. Available at: www.sages.org. Accessed October 1, 2013.
31. Rodriguez L, Rodriguez P, Gomez B, et al. Long-term results of electrical stimulation of the lower esophageal sphincter for the treatment of gastroesophageal reflux disease. Endoscopy 2013;45(8):595–604.

Gastroesophageal Reflux Disease and the Elderly

Sami R. Achem, MD, Kenneth R. DeVault, MD*

KEYWORDS

- Gastroesophageal reflux disease • Lower esophageal sphincter • Motility studies
- Barrett esophagus

KEY POINTS

- Gastroesophageal reflux disease (GERD) is a prevalent disorder in the elderly, and seems to be associated with more severe and advanced disease in a population that is growing in size in the United States.
- Changes in esophageal physiology predispose to more esophageal damage in older patients, as well as to a frequent disconnect between the type and severity of symptoms and severity of mucosal damage.
- Comorbidities make the diagnosis and treatment of GERD more challenging in aged patients, yet the treatment goals and approach are similar in older and younger patients.
- Older patients may be at increased risk of complications from reflux therapy, whether medical or surgical.

INTRODUCTION

Gastroesophageal reflux disease (GERD) is a common disorder affecting 20% of the United States population and 6% to 17% of the elderly.[1] GERD is not only common in the elderly, but when compared with younger counterparts, older patients have more intense patterns of abnormal acid contact time and advanced erosive disease.[2] The United States older population is growing and is at its highest level since 1900 according to the US Census Bureau. In 1900, there were fewer than 5 million Americans aged 65 and older. This rate increased to 35 million in 2000 and rose to more than 40 million by 2011, representing 13.8% of the total population.[3] By the year 2050, more than 20% of the United States population will be older than 65 years, and approximately 20 million individuals will be older than 85.[4]

There were about 1.5 million nursing home residents in 16,100 facilities according to the 2004 National Nursing Home Survey. The number of Americans needing long-term

The authors have no conflicts of interest to disclose in regard of this article.
Department of Medicine, Mayo Clinic College of Medicine, Jacksonville, FL, USA
* Corresponding author. Mayo Clinic, 4500 San Pablo Road, Jacksonville, FL 32224.
E-mail address: devault@mayo.edu

Gastroenterol Clin N Am 43 (2014) 147–160
http://dx.doi.org/10.1016/j.gtc.2013.11.004
0889-8553/14/$ – see front matter © 2014 Elsevier Inc. All rights reserved.

care is projected to double between 2000 and 2050.[5] A recent, retrospective cross-sectional study of almost 20,000 long-term care residents of nursing homes aged 65 years and older identified the 20 most common chronic conditions. GERD was the sixth most common disorder in the confined elderly, with 23% prevalence in men and women.[6] In summary, GERD is a prevalent disorder in the elderly, and seems to be associated with more severe and advanced disease in a population that is growing in size in the United States.

ESOPHAGEAL PHYSIOLOGY AND AGING

Aging of the esophagus has been associated with several important changes in esophageal physiology that predispose to both the prevalence and severity of GERD. These factors are summarized in **Box 1** and **Table 1**.

Structural Studies

In a rodent model, aging impairs the cholinergic nerve cell population in the stomach and intestines.[7] Studies of the animal or human esophagus appear scarce. In a study that evaluated the histology of the Auerbach plexus and esophageal smooth muscle in autopsy material from young and old subjects, the investigators found a significant decrease in ganglion cells per square centimeter ($P<.05$) and a heavier lymphocytic infiltration in comparison with younger counterparts.[8] This situation could potentially produce disorders similar to idiopathic achalasia and diffuse spasm. Pathologic changes seen in the esophagus with aging are similar to changes seen in patients with the more specific spastic esophageal motility disorders.[9]

Hiatal hernias are an important factor in the genesis of GERD, and their presence and size has been noted to partially correlate with the severity of mucosal damage from GERD. For example, hernias of 3 cm or larger may predispose to lower pressures in the lower esophageal sphincter (LES), greater acid exposure, and higher prevalence of erosive esophagitis.[10] Hernias are more common with increasing age, and were noted in 60% of patients older than 60 years.[11]

Esophageal Motility Studies

Lower esophageal sphincter

There is no clear relationship between basal LES pressure and aging.[12] When acid exposure and LES pressures were compared, LES pressure was lower with more severe acid exposure, but did not correlate with advancing age.[13] An additional study showed increased esophageal acid exposure with advancing age, and that these changes in acid exposure were associated with a decrease in both abdominal LES length and a weakening in esophageal motility.[14] Most studies seem to suggest that

---

Box 1
Potential factors that may predispose to GERD in older patients

Decreased salivary flow and bicarbonate secretion

Weakened and/or disordered esophageal motility

Weakened lower esophageal sphincter pressure

Hiatal hernia

Declining prevalence of *Helicobacter pylori* allows continued acid secretion into old age

Increased rates of obesity

Table 1
Potential factors that increase the severity of GERD in older patients

Factor	Mechanism/Notes
Weak UES pressure	Increased risk of aspiration
Decreased sensation	Increased risk of complications and delayed identification of disease
Poor primary and secondary peristalsis	Longer duration of acid exposure
Comorbidities (diabetes, medications, etc)	Increase acid exposure and/or increase severity of damage

LES pressure relates more to acid exposure and hiatal hernia than specifically to age. Transient LES relaxations (tLESR) are an important mechanism in GERD, and the authors are not aware of any studies looking at tLESR in older subjects in comparison with younger counterparts or controls.

Esophageal body

Much still remains to be learned about the effects of aging on esophageal physiology. In 1964, with the use of combined radiographic and esophageal manometric techniques, investigators coined the term presbyesophagus to suggest that elderly patients have a unique array of findings.[15] In 15 patients between 90 and 97 years old, they found evidence of nonpropulsive, often repetitive contractions and tertiary contractions in a pattern resembling esophageal spasm. Unfortunately, this study may have overestimated age-related deterioration because most of the patients were infirm with comorbidities that, by themselves, may explain the esophageal changes. Four were hospitalized patients, 4 had senile dementia, and 10 had evidence of diabetes and stroke or neuropathy.

Hollis and Castell[16] recruited 21 nonhospitalized elderly men (age 70–87 years) without evidence of diabetes, neuropathy, or dementia, and compared their basal and edrophonium-stimulated esophageal motility results with those of 11 men with no history of heartburn or dysphagia (age 19–27, mean 23 years). Their main finding was a decrease in basal esophageal pressures and a marked blunted cholinergic response ($P<.05$) in older patients (especially those >80 years) when compared with younger controls. The investigators concluded that disrupted muscle activity (rather than a neurologic process) was the explanation for the age-related differences. In another study, 10 normal subjects had repeated longitudinal studies over 8 years without evidence of deterioration in esophageal motility, but they were fairly young at the onset of the study (mean age 36, range 30–53 years).[17]

In a database of 562 patients undergoing manometry, 126 were noted to have aperistalsis. Detailed investigations were performed, which explained the aperistalsis in all patients except for a group of 26 elderly (>65 years) subjects. It was concluded that aging might be associated with deterioration of esophageal motility in these patients.[18] In 1979 a group in Barcelona, Spain published a study of 79 volunteers without obvious history of esophageal disease. Esophageal motility testing was done with a water-perfused system. To assess esophageal motility as a function of age, the 79 subjects were divided into 6 age groups ($\leq$25 [n = 26], 26–35 [n = 10], 36–45 [n = 10], 46–55 [n = 10], 56–65 [n = 10], >65 years [n = 13]). The results showed that LES pressure, upper esophageal sphincter (UES) pressure, and peristaltic wave amplitude and progression speed decrease with advancing age, whereas contractile wave duration and the proportion of nonperistaltic contractions increase.[19] A Brazilian study recruited 40 subjects from the community distributed by age (20 aged 20–30, 10 aged 50–60, and 10 aged 70–80 years), and performed esophageal manometry and scintigraphy. The investigators found abnormal peristalsis and impaired esophageal clearance to be more common in older volunteers.[20] In a population of 470 consecutive symptomatic esophageal patients (some with GERD and some with dysphagia and other symptoms referred for esophageal motility at a tertiary center), older patients (>75 years) tended to have more common abnormal motility (68.7%) when compared with their younger (<50 years) counterparts (45.7%).[12]

There are some motility data available from older patients who specifically have GERD. The effects of age on esophageal motility were recently reported in a study of 326 patients with symptoms and objective confirmation of GERD (erosions on esophagogastroduodenoscopy or abnormal pH). Subjects were grouped by decades. Whereas normal motility was observed in 87% of subjects aged 17 to 39 years, only 56% of those older than 70 had a normal study. Older age, but not GERD status, was also associated with lower esophageal amplitude of contraction. No age differences were noted in LES length or resting pressures, although, as expected for GERD subjects, LES resting pressures were lower on comparison with those without GERD (Fig. 1).[21] In an additional study of 349 consecutive patients undergoing motility and pH studies, the authors' group[22] found that when compared with younger subjects (age <40 years), older patients (>65 years) had a significantly lower percentage of normal swallow-induced peristalsis, and that peristaltic failure was associated with increased levels of esophageal acid exposure. These changes in esophageal motility were confirmed in a large (n = 1307) retrospective study.[14] Older GERD subjects had decreased abdominal LES length and esophageal motility. Age was associated with an increase in esophageal acid exposure, but the severity of reflux symptoms decreased with age.

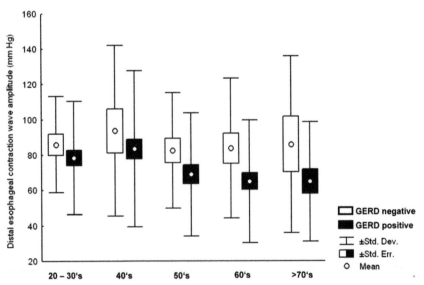

Fig. 1. Patients with GERD (GERD positive) were more likely to have lower distal esophageal amplitude, especially in the older age categories. (*From* Gutschow CA, Leers JM, Schröder W, et al. Effect of aging on esophageal motility in patients with and without GERD. Ger Med Sci 2011;9:Doc22.)

Upper esophageal sphincter dysfunction

Although not directly related to the pathophysiology of GERD, GERD-related aspiration into the airways is a potential cause of morbidity and mortality in the older patient.[23] Several studies have also identified several findings in this region of the esophagus. In 1990, a study of 10 elderly volunteers (age >60, range 62–79 years) and 10 younger adults (age <60, range 24–59 years) was completed with solid-state microtransducers. The investigators focused on UES physiology, and found that aging was associated with lower resting UES pressure and delayed UES relaxation, relative to the pharyngeal contraction peak.[24]

In a study of 67 healthy subjects aged 17 to 67 years, older subjects were found to have only marginally lower UES resting pressures but markedly elevated pharyngeal contraction pressures. Increasing age was associated with a reduction in duration of upper esophageal contractions and, for bread swallows, an increase in pharyngoesophageal wave velocity.[25] An additional, protective mechanism may also be affected with aging. Comparing 9 healthy young (26 ± 2 years) with 9 older subjects (77 ± 1 years), Ren and colleagues[26] noted significant differences in UES contractile reflex, showing this reflex to be impaired with age. This mechanism may be important in protecting the airway from aspiration of a refluxed bolus located in the proximal esophagus. Ongoing studies using high-resolution manometry may help to clarify the importance of the UES and proximal, striated muscle esophagus in reflux and other diseases.

Sensory Changes

Sensory changes in esophageal perception have also been noted, and may explain the concept that older patients often present with more advanced disease, but with symptoms similar to or milder than younger patients. When compared with younger control individuals (mean age 27, range 18–57 years), older subjects 65 years or greater (mean age 72.5, range 65–87 years) showed a decreased sensory perception to esophageal distension.[27] An acid perfusion study found that older patients with GERD were noted to have less severe symptoms and a longer lag time until the appearance of symptoms when compared with younger patients.[28]

Other Changes

Salivary bicarbonate is important in the neutralization of refluxed acid, and may tend to decrease with aging.[29] The relationship of aging and gastric acid secretion is somewhat complex. Historically it was suggested that older patients experience an age-related decrease in acid secretion, but this was likely related to *Helicobacter pylori* status.[30] Curing *H pylori* infection may actually increase reflux in some patients.[31] Because the prevalence of *H pylori* seems to be decreasing, more patients may retain their ability to secrete acid into old age. This continued acid secretion, when combined with some degree of peristaltic dysfunction, may lead to a greater risk for GERD and its complications. Other factors that have not been well studied in older patients include esophageal mucosa resistance, gastric emptying, and duodenogastric reflux.

Diabetes, Parkinson disease, Alzheimer disease, amyotrophic lateral sclerosis, and many other disorders increase in prevalence with aging, and thus may likely contribute to or are associated with GERD. Medication use is more common in older patients, and medications that may increase the risk of GERD include theophylline, nitrates, calcium antagonists, benzodiazepines, anticholinergics, antidepressants, lidocaine, and prostaglandins.[32] An increase in body weight with age may also predispose to GERD,[33] which is important because our older population is now more likely to be obese than in the past.[34]

AGE AND GERD PREVALENCE

The physiologic changes noted earlier likely predispose elderly patients to GERD, and an increased prevalence of GERD symptoms in elderly patients has been reported in some, but not all studies. The proportion of patients using antacids who are older than 50 years is greater than in patients younger than 50 (22% vs 9%).[35] On the other hand, in a random sample of 2200 residents of Olmsted County, Minnesota, aged 25 to 74 years, the overall prevalence of heartburn or acid regurgitation at least weekly was 20%, and no significant increase in prevalence occurred with age. The prevalence of heartburn declined with age although regurgitation did not.[1] This finding supports the concept of impaired sensory function with aging. A recent systematic review[36] found 9 population-based studies and 7 clinical studies on age-related prevalence and incidence. No increase in GERD symptom prevalence with age was noted, but aging was associated with more severe patterns of acid reflux and reflux esophagitis; symptoms associated with GERD become less severe and more nonspecific with aging (**Fig. 2**). The investigators concluded that "the real prevalence of GERD may well increase with age."[36]

CLINICAL PRESENTATION

In general, older patients with GERD have symptoms similar to those of younger patients, but complications and severe disease are more common, and include dysphagia, chest pain, and even GERD-related gastrointestinal bleeding. The severity

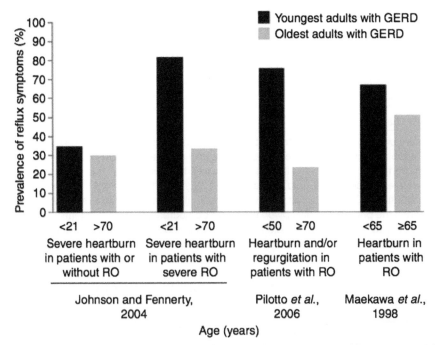

Fig. 2. Three studies in which severe heartburn was less common in older patients with erosive esophagitis (RO). (*From* Becher A, Dent J. Systematic review: aging and gastro-oesophageal reflux disease symptoms, esophageal function and reflux esophagitis. Aliment Pharmacol Ther 2011;33:450; with permission.)

of symptoms often does not correlate with the degree of esophageal damage and complications. In a study of 195 older patients with a mean age of 74 years, Raiha and colleagues[37] found heartburn to be absent in 50% of patients with esophagitis. Respiratory symptoms, dysphagia, and vomiting were common. Restrictive ventilatory defects[38] and lung parenchymal scars and pleural thickening,[39] in particular, are more common in older patients with increased acid exposure on 24-hour esophageal pH studies than in those with normal results. When symptoms were examined in more than 600 patients with erosive esophagitis, patients older than 65 years had fewer typical symptoms and more anorexia, weight loss, anemia, vomiting, and dysphagia (**Fig. 3**).[40] Typical symptoms were present in 40% of those older than 65 years, and in 65% of those older than 85. A questionnaire for the evaluation of upper gastrointestinal symptoms in the elderly (UGISQUE) has been developed and validated in elderly subjects with endoscopic diagnosis of reflux esophagitis, peptic

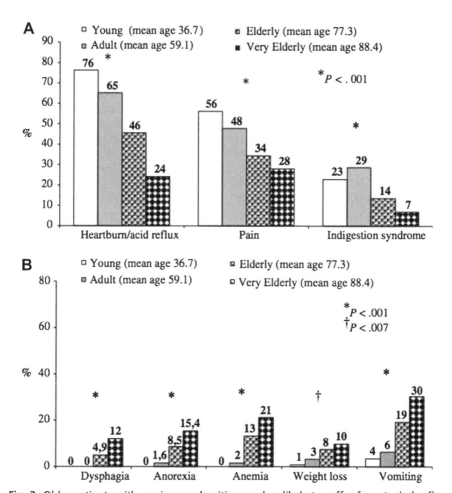

Fig. 3. Older patients with erosive esophagitis were less likely to suffer from typical reflux symptoms (A) and more likely to have atypical symptoms (B). (*From* Pilotto A, Franceschi M, Leandro G, et al. Clinical features of reflux esophagitis in older people: a study of 840 consecutive patients. J Am Geriatr Soc 2006;54:1539; with permission.)

ulcer, or erosive gastritis. The elderly patients had significantly higher rates of abdominal pain, reflux symptoms, indigestion syndrome, and bleeding, and also nonspecific symptoms, than subjects without endoscopic lesions.[41] In a retrospective study of almost 12,000 subjects undergoing detailed symptom evaluation and endoscopy,[42] severe esophagitis (Los Angeles grade C or D) became more common with aging while "severe" symptoms became less common (**Fig. 4**).

Complications

The risk of complications arising from GERD seems to be higher in older patients. Collen and colleagues[43] found erosive esophagitis in 81% of GERD patients older than 60, compared with 47% in those younger than 60 years. Barrett esophagus was also more common in older patients (25% vs 15%). A recent study from the Veterans Administration found more erosions, ulcers, and strictures in older patients, particularly older, white men.[44] In addition, in persons older than 80 years, esophagitis seems to account for a higher than expected proportion of patients with gastrointestinal bleeding.[45]

The incidence of Barrett esophagus clearly increases with age. Moreover, older patients with Barrett esophagus are less symptomatic than younger patients with Barrett esophagus.[46] Once Barrett is diagnosed in older patients, they usually are entered into a surveillance program. Many investigators have advocated an end to Barrett surveillance at some point as the patient ages, because of the unacceptable outcome of esophagectomy in older patients with high-grade dysplasia or cancer. The advent of less invasive, albeit still experimental approaches to dysplastic Barrett and early-stage adenocarcinoma, such as photodynamic therapy, catheter-based ablation, and localized mucosal resection, has resulted in older patients continuing with surveillance into advanced age. It is important to discuss the goals of Barrett surveillance with all patients. If the patient does not agree to endoscopic or surgical treatment of high-grade dysplasia or cancer, continued surveillance is unreasonable.

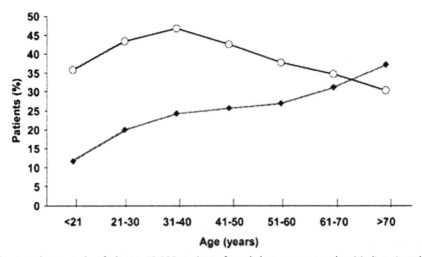

Fig. 4. A large study of almost 12,000 patients found that severe esophagitis (Los Angeles grade C or D) increased with age while severe symptoms tended to decrease. (*From* Johnson DA, Fennerty MB. Heartburn severity underestimates erosive esophagitis severity in elderly patients with gastroesophageal reflux disease. Gastroenterology 2004;126:662; with permission.)

TREATMENT
Medical Therapy

Although patients with GERD do not usually secrete more acid in comparison with controls, the treatment of GERD continues to usually involve acid suppression using either proton-pump inhibitors (PPIs) or H_2-receptor antagonists (H2RAs).

PPIs provide the greatest degree of acid suppression and are effective for most patients, regardless of age.[47] Some, but not all studies have suggested that older patients require more acid suppression than younger patients to heal erosive esophagitis.[48] On the other hand, a study comparing pantoprazole with nizatidine or placebo found that the PPI was superior in healing regardless of the age, and there were no age-related differences within each treatment arm.[49] Omeprazole has been available for many years and there have been several, additional PPI-related agents introduced in the past 20 years. Some of these have a slightly longer duration of action, but direct comparisons have required huge studies to find a small difference that may be of questionable clinical significance. Two agents (delayed-release dexlansoprazole and the bicarbonate/omeprazole combination) do not require administration before meals, which may be an advantage in some older patients.[50,51] The bicarbonate/omeprazole combination does contain a fair amount of sodium, which could produce issues in older patients with hypertension or fluid retention.

When using PPIs, particularly in older patients, several issues need to be taken into consideration. Plasma clearance of PPIs decreases with age, but no reduction in the dose of PPIs is necessary in older patients, even those with impaired renal or hepatic function.[52] Omeprazole and lansoprazole are metabolized by hepatic cytochrome P450 and may affect the metabolism of other drugs, but the effects been shown to be clinically insignificant with most agents.[53] Caution is still reasonable in older patients on multiple medications with similar metabolism, particularly if 1 of those medications has a narrow therapeutic window (eg, warfarin, phenytoin, diazepam, carbamazepine). Clopidogrel is a prodrug that is metabolized to its active form by the same cytochromes that metabolize most PPIs, and caution is advised when giving these medications together because in some patients combined therapy may decrease the efficacy of clopidogrel and lead to adverse vascular events.[54] This interaction has been extensively debated, and the most recently published guidelines for the treatment of GERD downplayed such an association.[55]

There may also be nutritional, metabolic, and infectious consequences of PPI therapy. Long-term use of a PPI may lead to a reduction in protein-bound vitamin B_{12} absorption,[56] but is unlikely to cause clinical B_{12} deficiency. Significant fat or carbohydrate malabsorption resulting from bacterial overgrowth is not likely with these agents.[57] The effect of PPI therapy on calcium absorption and subsequent bone density has become a topic of concern, especially among older patients, given a 2006 report suggesting an association between PPI therapy and hip fractures.[58] Other possible, but infrequent associations that should be remembered include an increased risk of community-acquired pneumonia and *Clostridium difficile* infection.[59] Another rare complication of PPI therapy is interstitial nephritis, which seems to be more common in older patients, with a mean age in one series of 78 years.[60] Finally, magnesium levels may also decrease when patients take PPIs for long periods.[61] Specific studies in older patients are lacking, but it would be easy to assume that these issues would be at least as common and perhaps more common in older patients.

Although PPIs have become the treatment of choice for GERD, some patients may be managed with H2RAs. For example, in maintenance trials PPIs are usually superior, but up to 50% of patients can be successfully stepped down from PPI therapy. In older patients, caution is required in using higher than standard doses of H2RAs. Changes in mental status have been described in older patients, particularly those with renal and liver dysfunction, with both cimetidine and ranitidine.[62] Cimetidine in particular may affect the metabolism of drugs by the hepatic cytochrome P450 system, including warfarin, theophylline, and benzodiazepines. In patients with renal insufficiency, the doses of all H2RAs may need to be reduced.[63] A study in African Americans suggested that older patients who were cognitively intact at baseline were more likely to develop cognitive impairment while on continuous H2RA treatment in comparison with nonusers.[64] Some patients, particularly those with infrequent symptoms, can be managed with as-needed H2RA or antacids. It is important to remember that antacids must be used with caution in the elderly because of the potential risk of salt overload, constipation, diarrhea, and the possible interference with the absorption of other drugs.

The best therapy for GERD would prevent reflux without necessarily decreasing acid secretion using a motility agent. Unfortunately, the lack of efficacy and high rate of side effects with these agents makes the routine use of promotility agents for the treatment of GERD in this (or any) population problematic and often inappropriate. Metoclopramide is a dopamine antagonist that increases LES pressure and improves gastric emptying,[65] but must be used with great caution in older patients because of side effects in up to one-third of patients, including muscle tremors, spasms, agitation, anxiety, insomnia, drowsiness, and even frank confusion or tardive dyskinesia.[66] This problem has led regulatory agencies in the United States to place a black-box warning on metoclopramide. Domperidone is a similar agent, but with little to no central nervous system (CNS) interactions, although it has not been proved to be very effective in GERD and is not routinely available in the United States. Cisapride had some degree of efficacy in mild GERD, but can cause cardiac arrhythmias and has been removed from the market in most, if not all countries. Bethanechol, which increases resting LES pressure, is rarely used and is associated with various side effects, including urinary frequency, abdominal pain, blurred vision, and worsening glaucoma, all of which are more likely in an older patient. Agents designed to function like bethanechol, but with fewer CNS side effects, have thus far not reached the market because of poor efficacy, side effects, or both.

It is clear that acid-suppressing agents are extensively used throughout the world, and there are data suggesting substantial overuse and inappropriate use. For example, in a study looking at preadmission and postadmission medication use in a group of older, hospitalized patients,[67] PPIs were listed in 40% of admitted patients and no accepted indication was identifiable in 66% of these patients. PPIs (and any medication) should be discontinued when there is no indication for their use, particularly when it is not having an appreciable effect on the symptoms being treated.

Surgical Therapy

Surgery can be performed successfully in older patients who are reasonable operative risks, but should be avoided in patients with concomitant medical problems that make such surgery hazardous. When a group of surgical patients older than 70 years was compared with a group younger than 60, preoperative and postoperative reflux symptom scores were lower in the older patients, but all other outcomes and complications were similar between the two groups (with the exception of postoperative dysphagia, which was actually less common in the older patients).[68] An additional series also reported similar outcomes, with the only significant findings being more atypical symptoms and more impaired preoperative motility in the older patients.[69] Large, paraesophageal hernias are an additional surgical problem in the older patient with

GERD, although most investigators suggest that these only be repaired when they are symptomatic or producing complications. Laparoscopic repair of large and/or complicated hernias is technically challenging and is also associated with higher complication and recurrence rates, but can be successful even in very old patients.[70] Regardless of the type of hernia (standard hiatal, paraesophageal, or mixed), older patients are at risk for weak peristalsis and postoperative dysphagia. The authors continue to use the preoperative esophageal motility study to guide surgery, particularly in older patients. There are several new approaches to GERD (both endoscopic and laparoscopic) in development, but there are no data from older patients.

SUMMARY

Older patients have changes in their esophageal physiology that predispose to more severe forms of GERD, and also may mask symptoms and delay or prevent health care providers from recognizing esophageal damage from refluxed acid, including esophagitis and Barrett esophagus. Older patients are at increased risk for GERD complications and also have frequent atypical presentations. Comorbidities make the diagnosis and treatment of GERD more challenging in aged patients. The treatment goals and approach are similar for older and younger patients. Therapy can include chronic PPI therapy and antireflux surgery in selected patients, but some can be managed with lifestyle changes and less aggressive therapy. Older patients may be at increased risk of complications from reflux therapy, whether medical or surgical.

REFERENCES

1. Locke GR, Talley NJ, Fett SL, et al. Prevalence and clinical spectrum of gastroesophageal reflux: a population-based study in Olmstead County, Minnesota. Gastroenterology 1997;112:1448–56.
2. Zhu H, Pace F, Sangaletti O, et al. Features of symptomatic gastroesophageal reflux in elderly patients. Scand J Gastroenterol 1993;28:235–8.
3. Department of Health and Human Services. A profile of older Americans: 2011. Available at: http://www.aoa.gov/Aging_Statistics/Profile/2011/docs/2011profile.pdf.
4. Greenwald DA. Aging, the gastrointestinal tract, and risk of acid-related disease. Am J Med 2004;117:8S–13S.
5. US Department of Health and Human Services and US Department of Labor. The future supply of long-term care workers in relation to the aging baby boom generation: report to Congress. Washington, DC: U.S. Government Printing Office; 2003. Available at: http://aspe.hhs.gov/daltcp/reports/ltcwork.htm. Accessed December 1, 2013.
6. Moore KL, Boscardin WJ, Steinman MA, et al. Age and sex variation in prevalence of chronic medical conditions in older residents of U.S. nursing homes. J Am Geriatr Soc 2012;60:756–64.
7. Phillips RJ, Kieffer EJ, Powley TL. Aging of the myenteric plexus: neuronal loss is specific to cholinergic neurons. Auton Neurosci 2003;106:69–83.
8. Eckardt VF, LeCompte PM. Esophageal ganglia and smooth muscle in the elderly. Am J Dig Dis 1978;23:443–8.
9. Adams CW, Brain RH, Trounce JR. Ganglion cells in achalasia of the cardia. Virchows Arch A Pathol Anat Histol 1976;372:75–9.
10. Patti MG, Goldberg HI, Arcerito M, et al. Hiatal hernia size affects lower esophageal sphincter function, esophageal acid exposure, and the degree of mucosal injury. Am J Surg 1996;171:182–6.

11. Khajanchee YS, Urbach DR, Butler N, et al. Laparoscopic antireflux surgery in the elderly. Surg Endosc 2002;16:25–30.
12. Richter JE, Wu WC, Johns DN, et al. Esophageal manometry in 95 healthy adult volunteers. Variability of pressures with age and frequency of "abnormal" contractions. Dig Dis Sci 1987;32:583–92.
13. Ribeiro AC, Klingler PJ, Hinder RA, et al. Esophageal manometry: a comparison of findings in younger and older patients. Am J Gastroenterol 1998;93:706–10.
14. Lee J, Anggiansha A, Anggiansah R, et al. Effects of age on the gastroesophageal junction, esophageal motility, and reflux disease. Clin Gastroenterol Hepatol 2007;5:1392–8.
15. Soergel KH, Zboralske FF, Amberg JR. Presbyesophagus: esophageal motility in nonagenarians. J Clin Invest 1964;43:1472–9.
16. Hollis JB, Castell DO. Esophageal function in elderly man. A new look at "presbyesophagus". Ann Intern Med 1974;80:371–4.
17. Kruse-Andersen S, Wallin L, Madsen T. The influence of age on esophageal acid defense mechanisms and spontaneous acid gastroesophageal reflux. Am J Gastroenterol 1988;83:637–9.
18. Meshkinpour H, Haghighat P, Dutton C. Clinical spectrum of esophageal aperistalsis in the elderly. Am J Gastroenterol 1994;89:1480–3.
19. Grande L, Lacima G, Ros E, et al. Deterioration of esophageal motility with age: a manometric study of 79 healthy subjects. Am J Gastroenterol 1999;94:1795–801.
20. Ferriolli E, Oliveira RB, Matsuda NM, et al. Aging, esophageal motility, and gastroesophageal reflux. J Am Geriatr Soc 1998;46:1534–7.
21. Gutschow CA, Leers JM, Schröder W, et al. Effect of aging on esophageal motility in patients with and without GERD. Ger Med Sci 2011;9:Doc22.
22. Achem AC, Achem SR, Stark ME, et al. Failure of esophageal peristalsis in older patients: association with esophageal acid exposure. Am J Gastroenterol 2003; 98:35–9.
23. Marik PE, Kaplan D. Aspiration pneumonia and dysphagia in the elderly. Chest 2003;124:328–36.
24. Fulp SR, Dalton CB, Castell JA, et al. Aging-related alterations in human upper esophageal sphincter function. Am J Gastroenterol 1990;85:1569–72.
25. Wilson JA, Pryde A, Macintyre CC, et al. The effects of age, sex, and smoking on normal pharyngoesophageal motility. Am J Gastroenterol 1990;85:686–91.
26. Ren J, Xie P, Lang IM, et al. Deterioration of the pharyngo-UES contractile reflex in the elderly. Laryngoscope 2000;110:1563–6.
27. Lasch H, Castell DO, Castell JA. Evidence for diminished visceral pain with aging: studies using graded intraesophageal balloon distension. Am J Physiol 1997;272:G1–3.
28. Fass R, Pulliam G, Johnson C, et al. Symptom severity and oesophageal chemosensitivity to acid in older and young patients with gastro-oesophageal reflux. Age Ageing 2000;29:125–30.
29. Sonnenberg A, Steinkamp U, Weise A, et al. Salivary secretion in reflux esophagitis. Gastroenterology 1982;83:889–95.
30. Hurwitz A, Brady DA, Schaal SE, et al. Gastric acidity in older adults. JAMA 1997;278:659–62.
31. Labenz J, Blum AL, Bayerdorffer E, et al. Curing *Helicobacter pylori* infection in patients with duodenal ulcer may provoke reflux esophagitis. Gastroenterology 1997;112:1442–7.
32. Richter JE, Castell DO. Gastroesophageal reflex. Pathogenesis, diagnosis, and therapy. Ann Intern Med 1982;97:93–103.

33. Wajed SA, Streets CG, Bremner CG, et al. Elevated body mass disrupts the barrier to gastroesophageal reflux. Arch Surg 2001;136:1014–9.
34. Arterburn DE, Crane PK, Sullivan SD. The coming epidemic of obesity in elderly Americans. J Am Geriatr Soc 2004;52:1907–12.
35. Gallup Organization. A Gallup survey on heartburn across America. Princeton (NJ): Gallup Organization; 1988.
36. Becher A, Dent J. Systematic review: ageing and gastro-oesophageal reflux disease symptoms, oesophageal function and reflux oesophagitis. Aliment Pharmacol Ther 2011;33:442–54.
37. Raiha I, Hietanen E, Sourander L. Symptoms of gastro-oesophageal reflux disease in elderly people. Age Ageing 1991;20:365–70.
38. Raiha IJ, Ivaska K, Sourander LB. Pulmonary function in gastro-oesophageal reflux disease of elderly people. Age Ageing 1992;21:368–73.
39. Raiha I, Manner R, Hietanen E, et al. Radiographic pulmonary changes of gastro-oesophageal reflux disease in elderly patients. Age Ageing 1992;21:250–5.
40. Pilotto A, Franceschi M, Leandro G, et al. Clinical features of reflux esophagitis in older people: a study of 840 consecutive patients. J Am Geriatr Soc 2006;54:1537–42.
41. Pilotto A, Maggi S, Noale M, et al. Development and validation of a new questionnaire for the evaluation of upper gastrointestinal symptoms in the elderly population: a multicenter study. J Gerontol A Biol Sci Med Sci 2010;65:174–8.
42. Johnson DA, Fennerty MB. Heartburn severity underestimates erosive esophagitis severity in elderly patients with gastroesophageal reflux disease. Gastroenterology 2004;126:660–4.
43. Collen MJ, Abdulian JD, Chen YK. Gastroesophageal reflux disease in the elderly: more severe disease that requires aggressive therapy. Am J Gastroenterol 1995;90:1053–7.
44. El-Serag HB, Sonnenberg A. Associations between different forms of gastro-oesophageal reflux disease. Gut 1997;41:594–9.
45. Zimmerman J, Shohat V, Tsvang E, et al. Esophagitis is a major cause of upper gastrointestinal hemorrhage in the elderly. Scand J Gastroenterol 1997;32:906–9.
46. Grade A, Pulliam G, Johnson C, et al. Reduced chemoreceptor sensitivity in patients with Barrett's esophagus may be related to age and not to the presence of Barrett's epithelium. Am J Gastroenterol 1997;92:2040–3.
47. Hetzel DJ, Dent J, Reed WD, et al. Healing and relapse of severe peptic esophagitis after treatment with omeprazole. Gastroenterology 1988;95:903–12.
48. Garnett WR, Garabedian-Ruffalo SM. Identification, diagnosis, and treatment of acid-related diseases in the elderly: implications for long-term care. Pharmacotherapy 1997;17:938–58.
49. DeVault KR, Morgenstern DM, Lynn RB, et al. Effect of pantoprazole in older patients with erosive esophagitis. Dis Esophagus 2007;20:411–5.
50. Lee RD, Vakily M, Mulford D, et al. Clinical trial: the effect and timing of food on the pharmacokinetics and pharmacology of dexlansoprazole MR, a novel dual delayed release formulation of a proton pump inhibitor-evidence for dosing flexibility. Aliment Pharmacol Ther 2009;29:824–33.
51. Katz PO, Koch FK, Ballard ED, et al. Comparison of the effects of immediate-release omeprazole oral suspension, delayed-release lansoprazole capsules and delayed-release esomeprazole capsules on nocturnal gastric acidity after bedtime. Aliment Pharmacol Ther 2007;25:197–205.

52. McTavish D, Buckley MM, Heel RC. Omeprazole. An updated review of its pharmacology and therapeutic use in acid-related disorders. Drugs 1991;42:138–70.
53. Andersson T. Pharmacokinetics, metabolism and interactions of acid pump inhibitors. Focus on omeprazole, lansoprazole and pantoprazole. Clin Pharmacokinet 1996;31:9–28.
54. Laine L, Hennekens C. Proton pump inhibitor and clopidogrel interaction: fact or fiction? Am J Gastroenterol 2010;105:34–41.
55. Katz PO, Gerson LB, Vela M. Guidelines for the diagnosis and management of gastroesophageal reflux disease. Am J Gastroenterol 2013;108(3):308–28.
56. Saltzman JR, Kemp JA, Golner BB, et al. Effect of hypochlorhydria due to omeprazole treatment or atrophic gastritis on protein-bound vitamin B12 absorption. J Am Coll Nutr 1994;13:584–91.
57. Saltzman JR, Kowdley KV, Pedrosa MC, et al. Bacterial overgrowth without clinical malabsorption in elderly hypochlorhydric subjects. Gastroenterology 1994; 106:615–23.
58. Yang YX, Lewis JD, Epstein S, et al. Long-term proton pump inhibitor therapy and risk of hip fracture. JAMA 2006;296:2947–53.
59. DeVault KR, Talley NJ. Insights into the future of gastric acid suppression. Nat Rev Gastroenterol Hepatol 2009;6(9):524–32.
60. Sierra F, Suarez M, Rey M, et al. Systematic review: proton pump inhibitor-associated acute interstitial nephritis. Aliment Pharmacol Ther 2007;26:545–53.
61. Cundy T, Dissanayake A. Severe hypomagnesaemia in long-term users of proton-pump inhibitors. Clin Endocrinol 2008;69:338–41.
62. Lipsy RJ, Fennerty B, Fagan TC. Clinical review of histamine2 receptor antagonists. Arch Intern Med 1990;150:745–51.
63. Hatlebakk JG, Berstad A. Pharmacokinetic optimisation in the treatment of gastro-oesophageal reflux disease. Clin Pharmacokinet 1996;31:386–406.
64. Boustani M, Hall KS, Lane KA, et al. The association between cognition and histamine-2 receptor antagonists in African Americans. J Am Geriatr Soc 2007;55:1248–53.
65. Lieberman DA, Keeffe EB. Treatment of severe reflux esophagitis with cimetidine and metoclopramide. Ann Intern Med 1986;104:21–6.
66. Verlinden M. Review article: a role for gastrointestinal prokinetic agents in the treatment of reflux oesophagitis? Aliment Pharmacol Ther 1989;3:113–31.
67. Pasina L, Hobili A, Tettamanti M, et al. Prevalence and appropriateness of drug prescriptions for peptic ulcer and gastro-oesophageal reflux disease in a cohort of hospitalized elderly. Eur J Intern Med 2011;22:205–10.
68. Cowgill SM, Arnaoutakis D, Villadolid D, et al. Results after laparoscopic fundoplication: does age matter? Am Surg 2006;72:448–83.
69. Pizza F, Rossetti G, Limongelli P, et al. Influence of age on outcome of total laparoscopic fundoplication for gastroesophageal reflux disease. World J Gastroenterol 2007;13:740–7.
70. Gupta A, Change D, Steele KE, et al. Looking beyond age and co-morbidities as predictors of outcome in paraesophageal hernia repair. J Gastrointest Surg 2008;12:2119–24.

Obesity and GERD

Paul Chang, MD, Frank Friedenberg, MD, MS (Epi)*

KEYWORDS

- Obesity • Gastroesophageal reflux disease • Barrett esophagus • Waist-to-hip ratio
- Adiponectin • Leptin

KEY POINTS

- The prevalence of obesity and gastroesophageal reflux disease (GERD) has increased substantially in the past 30 years.
- Central adiposity, measured as the waist-to-hip ratio, is more closely associated with GERD complications than measures of overall obesity such as body mass index.
- Visceral adipose tissue is metabolically active and secretes adipokines along with inflammatory cytokines that may predispose to complications of GERD such as Barrett esophagus and esophageal carcinoma.

INTRODUCTION
Disease Description

The typical manifestations of gastroesophageal reflux disease (GERD) are heartburn and/or regurgitation. GERD can be further classified into erosive GERD and nonerosive GERD based on endoscopic appearance of esophageal mucosa. The term "atypical GERD" is used in situations where the predominant symptoms are extraesophageal such as cough, laryngitis, and asthma.[1] GERD is a common disorder with a prevalence of approximately 20% in the United States.[2] The recognized sequelae of GERD include Barrett esophagus (BE) and esophageal adenocarcinoma. Obesity, defined as a body mass index (BMI) greater than or equal to 30, is common in the Western world and is increasing in other parts of the world, particularly Asia. Epidemiologic data demonstrate that overall obesity (typically measured as BMI kg/m^2) is a risk factor for both GERD and esophageal adenocarcinoma.[3] There is evidence that central abdominal obesity, as opposed to an elevated BMI, is the most important factor associated with BE (**Table 1**).[4]

PREVALENCE/INCIDENCE

A systematic review estimated the prevalence of GERD in the United States at 18.1% to 27.8%.[2] El-Serag and others in their systematic review divided studies on the

Section of Gastroenterology, Temple University School of Medicine, Philadelphia, PA, USA
* Corresponding author. Temple University Hospital, Parkinson Pavilion, 8th Floor, 3401 North Broad Street, Philadelphia, PA 19140.
E-mail address: friedfk@tuhs.temple.edu

Gastroenterol Clin N Am 43 (2014) 161–173
http://dx.doi.org/10.1016/j.gtc.2013.11.009
0889-8553/14/$ – see front matter © 2014 Elsevier Inc. All rights reserved.

| Table 1 |
Risk factors for GERD
Obesity
Caffeine intake
Spicy foods
Tobacco
Pregnancy
Alcohol
Recumbent position
Connective tissue disorders
Hiatal hernia
Decreased LES tone
Zollinger-Ellison syndrome
Post-prandial supination

prevalence of GERD into 4 temporal categories. Relative to pre-1995, the rate ratio for GERD prevalence was 1.45 for the period 1995 to 1999, 1.46 for 2000 to 2004, and 1.51 for 2005 to 2009. Obesity is an even more common health issue in the United States. Data from the 2009–2010 National Health and Examination Survey estimate a prevalence of 35.5% for men and 35.8% for women, which is not significantly changed compared with the period 2003 to 2008.[5] Previous trends showed that the prevalence of obesity was increasing in America but the trend may be beginning to level.

Cross-sectional epidemiologic studies have demonstrated a higher prevalence of GERD in obese individuals compared with the nonobese. Jacobsen and colleagues[6] used a supplemental GERD questionnaire added to the Nurses' Health Study to show that subjects who reported at least weekly symptoms had a near linear increase in the adjusted odds ratio (OR) for reflux symptoms for each BMI strata. A similar link was seen in the results from the 80,110 insurance members from the Kaiser Permanente Multi-Phasic Health Check-Up cohort.[7] The association between BMI and GERD was stronger among whites compared with black members, with ORs of 1.58 and 1.33, respectively. When controlling for abdominal diameter the ORs were 1.39 and 1.15, respectively.

Smaller studies have confirmed the link between obesity and GERD. El-Serag and others interviewed 453 hospital employees and found that 26% had weekly heartburn or regurgitation symptoms.[8] Subjects were offered endoscopy and 196 agreed, and they found that increasing levels of obesity were associated with a greater likelihood of GERD and esophagitis. The proportion of subjects with GERD symptoms were 23.3%, 26.7%, and 50% for BMI groups <25, 25–30, and >30, respectively. Prevalence rates for erosive esophagitis (EE) were 12.5%, 29.8%, and 26.9%. Two small cohort studies from Olmstead County, MN have also evaluated the relationship between obesity and GERD. The first study identified obesity as a risk factor for the initial development of GERD as well as the persistence of symptoms.[9] The second study found that BMI was associated with GERD (OR = 1.9) independent of diet and energy expenditure.[10]

The effect of weight change on GERD symptoms has been studied. Jacobson and colleagues[6] studied select individuals from the Nurses' Health Study and found that an increase of BMI by more than 3.5 kg/m^2 when compared with no weight change was associated with an increase risk of frequent symptoms of reflux.

WORLD-WIDE INCIDENCE RATES

The prevalence of obesity is somewhat lower outside of the United States. The European Prospective Investigation into Cancer and Nutrition study estimated the prevalence of obesity was 17% in 2005, which increased from 13% in 1998.[11] Based on a systematic review, the prevalence rate of GERD in Europe was estimated to be 15% for the period 2005 to 2009. Similar to the trend seen in the United States, this prevalence rate is significantly higher than the rate before 1995.[2] The epidemiologic relationship between obesity and GERD has been observed in Europe as well. The German National Health Interview and Examination Survey found the OR for GERD to be 1.8 for overweight and 2.6 for obese individuals.[12] In England, the Bristol Helicobacter Project found that obese individuals had an OR of 2.91 for heartburn and an OR of 2.23 for regurgitation.[13] A telephone survey in Spain of 2500 subjects revealed that obese individuals had an OR of 1.74 for GERD symptoms. It was also noted that patients with GERD symptoms for more than 10 years were more likely to be obese (OR = 1.92).[14] This group also found that a weight gain of more than 5 kg in the past year demonstrated a 2.7-fold higher risk of new GERD symptoms.[15] In Norway, Nilsson and colleagues[16] conducted nationwide surveys during the periods 1984 to 1986 (N = 74,599) and 1995 to 1997 (N = 65,363). They found that for severely obese men (BMI>35 kg/m^2) the OR for GERD was 3.3, whereas the OR for severely obese women was 6.3. A link showing an association between estrogen levels and GERD was observed. Premenopausal women and those who were post-menopausal but taking hormone replacement therapy were at an increased risk for GERD relative to untreated post-menopausal women.

A relationship between obesity and GERD has been seen in Asia. Kang and colleagues[17] studied 2457 subjects who underwent upper endoscopy in Korea. They found a relationship between higher strata of BMI and the presence of EE. In Shanghai, a nested case-control study found an association between obesity and dwelling in an urban environment with GERD.[18]

Studies that have failed to identify a relationship between GERD and obesity have also been reported. A study of 820 subjects from Sweden showed that those who had been overweight or obese had an adjusted OR of 0.99 for GERD. They also found no association between obesity and severity of reflux symptoms.[19] Similarly, a prospective cohort study in Olmsted, MN of 607 individuals surveyed more than 10.5 years did not find an association with GERD symptoms and weight loss of greater than 10 pounds.[9]

In summary, the preponderance of population-based studies supports the association between obesity and GERD reflux. The association has been demonstrated in the United States where obesity rates are the highest and has also been seen in Europe and Eastern Asia (**Fig. 1**). Shortcomings of these studies are that they primarily relied on self-reported height and weight to calculate BMI and did not look specifically at abdominal obesity. There appears to be a dose response as well with increasing levels of obesity associated with higher prevalence rates. Weight loss has not been consistently associated with amelioration of symptoms at a population level.

CLINICAL CORRELATION
Complications of GERD

Long-term complications of GERD such as EE, BE, and esophageal adenocarcinoma have been associated with obesity. In a large endoscopic study, El-Serag reported that relative to those with no erosions, those with EE were more likely to be overweight or obese.[8] A similar association was seen in Korea where Lee and colleagues[29] did an endoscopy study in Korea studying 3000 participants. They found that obese individuals compared to normal weight subjects had an OR of 3.3 for EE. A meta-analysis by Hampel and colleagues[30] confirmed the association with increasing levels of obesity and esophageal mucosal injury.

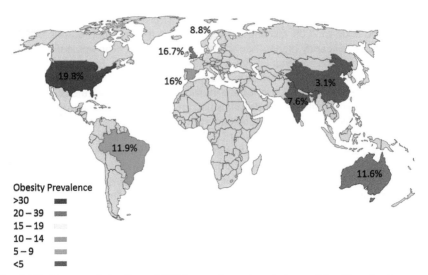

Fig. 1. World map of obesity and GERD prevalence in select countries. The obesity prevalence coded by the color key. The percentages indicate the GERD prevalence. (*Data from* Refs.[2,5,20–28])

Associations of BE and obesity have been demonstrated by Stein and colleagues[31] who established that for each 5-unit increase in BMI, the risk of BE increased by 35%. Abdominal obesity ("central obesity") has been shown to be a more specific risk factor for BE. Corley and colleagues,[32] using data from the Kaiser Permanente database, found that a larger abdominal circumference (measured at the iliac crest with the abdomen relaxed), independent of BMI, was associated with BE. Edelstein and colleagues[33] found that for individuals in the highest category of waist-to-hip ratio the adjusted OR for BE was 1.9 and 4.1 for long-segment BE. Rubenstein and colleagues[34] found that abdominal obesity as measured by waist circumference increased the risk of EE and BE, whereas gluteofemoral obesity was protective. Finally, El-Serag used abdominal computed tomographic imaging to demonstrate that greater amounts of visceral adipose tissue but not subcutaneous adipose tissue conferred a significantly increased risk for BE.[4]

Not all studies have demonstrated an association between obesity and BE. An Australian study found that BMI was not an independent risk factor for BE.[35] A study in Canada by Veugelers and colleagues[36] also did not show an association between obesity and BE. They did, however, find an association of BMI with esophageal adenocarcinoma.

The incidence of esophageal adenocarcinoma has been rising in the United States.[37] From 1975 to 2001, the incidence of esophageal adenocarcinoma has increased approximately 6-fold. There are several studies that have examined the relationship between obesity and esophageal adenocarcinoma. In 1998, a National Cancer Institute study by Chow and colleagues[38] found an association between increasing strata of BMI and esophageal cancer, specifically among younger nonsmoking individuals. A Swedish study identified obesity with an OR of 16.2 for the development of adenocarcinoma compared with the leanest individuals (BMI<22 kg/m^2). A recently pooled analysis from 12 world-wide epidemiologic studies showed that patients with a BMI greater than or equal to 40 compared with nonoverweight patients had an OR of 4.76 for esophageal adenocarcinoma.[39] Engel and colleagues[40] found that the population attributable risk (proportion of occurrences in the population that may be preventable if a factor were totally eliminated) for body weight (using BMI<23.1 as the control group) increased steadily from 5.4% (BMI = 23.2–25.1) to 21.3% (BMI = 27.3–40.1).

Pathophysiology

Several physiologic abnormalities that could lead to prolonged esophageal acid exposure have been found to occur more frequently in obese compared with normal weight individuals. Many of these disturbances have been identified in the severely obese (BMI>35) before bariatric surgery and may not apply to those with lesser degrees of obesity. For example, esophageal manometry before bariatric surgery has revealed that many patients have a motility disorder. In a study of 345 patients, 25.6% of patients had abnormal manometry. The most common abnormal findings were nutcracker esophagus and nonspecific motility disorder.[41] Other studies in severely obese subjects revealed similar findings, with nonspecific motility disorder, nutcracker esophagus, and hypotensive lower esophageal sphincter (LES) as the most common manometric abnormalities.[42,43] Interestingly, most of these patients were asymptomatic.

Studies looking specifically at prebariatric surgical patients with symptoms of GERD excluding asymptomatic patients have also been reported. Hong and colleagues[44] studied 61 patients and 32.8% had abnormal manometry, most commonly nonspecific esophageal motor disorder. Another study using manometry, 24-hour pH measurement, and impedance grouped patients into 3 groups. Group 1 (control group) had 10 normal-weight asymptomatic subjects, group 2 had 22 nonobese GERD patients, and group 3 consisted of 22 obese GERD patients. All group 1 patients had normal esophageal acid exposure, motility, and bolus transit. From group 2 there were 5 patients with abnormal manometry, 2 with ineffective esophageal motility, 2 with nutcracker esophagus, and 1 with hypertensive LES (>50 mm Hg). Group 3 also had 5 patients with abnormal manometry, including 2 with ineffective esophageal motility, 2 with nutcracker esophagus, and 1 with diffuse esophageal spasm. The only difference between the obese and nonobese GERD subjects was that obese patients had fewer episodes of complete bolus transit (as measured by impedance) compared with the nonobese, 66% versus 88% $P = .01$.[45]

A hypotensive LES, defined as basal pressure less than 10 mm Hg, is clearly a predisposing factor for GERD. Studies examining the relationship between LES pressure and BMI have been performed, although the results are inconsistent. One study examined 64 consecutive patients and divided subjects into 3 groups. Group A had 23 subjects with a BMI less than 25, group B had 25 subjects with a BMI between 25 and 30, and group C had 16 subjects with a BMI >30. The investigators observed a strong inverse relationship between BMI and LES pressure ($P<.001$).[46]

Transient relaxations of the lower esophageal sphincter (TRLES) have been observed to be more common in patients with obesity. The main stimulus for TRLES is gastric distension, particularly in the fundus.[47,48] A study by Wu and colleagues[49] divided subjects into 3 groups, 28 obese, 28 overweight, and 28 normal subjects. These individuals were studied with upper endoscopy, manometry, and pH recordings. The overweight and obese groups were found to have significantly higher rates of TRLES during the 2-hour postprandial period (obese group 17.3, overweight 3.8, normal 2.1 episodes per hour; $P<.001$). Total distal esophageal acid exposure as well as the proportion of TRLES accompanied by acid reflux was also greater in the obese and overweight groups.

The presence of a hiatal hernia has also been associated with obesity. Suter and colleagues[41] studied morbidly obese patients with history of reflux symptoms with upper endoscopy, 24-hour pH monitoring, and manometry. They observed that of

345 subjects approximately half had a hiatal hernia. Furthermore, patients with a hiatal hernia were more likely to have esophagitis compared with those without a hiatal hernia. Pandolfino and colleagues[50] subsequently reported that obese patients have a pressure gradient along the esophagogastric junction that supported the development of a hiatal hernia.

Abdominal obesity likely increases intra-abdominal pressure due to transmission of gravitational force of the adipose tissue to the abdominal cavity. Lambert and colleagues[51] studied morbidly obese patients with a urinary catheter as a surrogate for intra-abdominal pressure and found that obese patients compared with nonobese patients had higher intra-abdominal pressures. This relationship between obesity and elevated intra-abdominal/intragastric pressures has been confirmed by others with use of intragastric manometry.[52,53]

Gastric volume and motor abnormalities have been proposed as other mechanisms for GERD in obese individuals. Multiple studies have found that the capacitance of gastric contents in obese subjects is larger compared with lean individuals.[54,55] Whether the greater volume of contents leads to increased GERD is not known. It has also been theorized that obese individuals may have delayed gastric emptying due to neuronal or humoral mechanisms.[56–58] Buchholz and colleagues[59] using standardized scintigraphic gastric emptying studies showed no difference in gastric emptying in obese and nonobese patients. Retention percentages at 1 hour and 4 hours were 48% and 47% and 1.7% and 1.1%, respectively.

The link between obesity and esophageal neoplasia may be via altered secretion of adipokines such as adiponectin and leptin. Adiponectin is a protein that has antiinflammatory and immunomodulatory functions and stimulates apoptosis.[60] Secretion of adiponectin decreases with obesity. Rubenstein and colleagues[61] found an inverse association between plasma adiponectin levels and the presence of BE in a case-control study. In a separate study, this group found that levels of the low molecular weight subtype of adiponectin were inversely associated with the risk of BE.[62] In contrast to the inverse relationship seen between obesity and adiponectin, leptin levels correlate directly with obesity.[63] Leptin is secreted by adipocytes and gastric chief cells and has been shown to have mitogenic properties and induce proliferation in several human cell lines including esophageal cancer cells.[64] Kendall and colleagues[65] found that male subjects with BE had higher levels of plasma leptin relative to healthy controls. Those with a leptin level in the highest quartile had an OR of 3.3 for the presence of BE. The link between BE and central obesity (rather than BMI) may be partially explained by the fact that leptin reaches very high values in central obesity (**Figs. 2** and **3**).

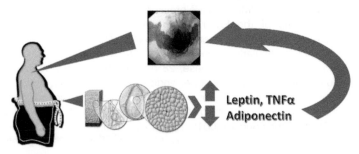

Fig. 2. Mechanism of increased abdominal obesity leading to BE. The increased adipose tissue leads to increases in leptin and tumor necrosis factor α, which have been linked to a higher risk of BE. Increased adipose tissue has also been inversely linked with adiponectin levels, which are protective for the development of BE.

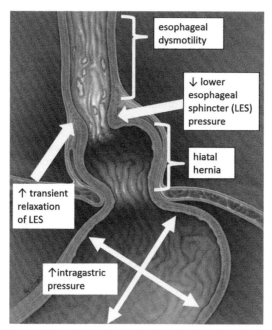

Fig. 3. Summary of potential pathogenic mechanisms in the obese leading to GERD.

Weight Loss and GERD

In Norway, the HUNT 3 study surveyed 44,997 subjects from 2006 to 2009 and found that weight loss was dose-dependently associated with a reduction of symptoms.[66] A prospective cohort study of 332 obese adults enrolled in a structured weight loss program was performed by Singh and colleagues.[67] Mean weight loss was 13 kg and the prevalence of GERD decreased from 37% to 15% with 81% of subjects experiencing a reduction in symptom scores. Fraser-Moodie and colleagues[68] observed 34 patients who had GERD and a BMI greater than 23. Patients were given dietary advice (not a structured weight loss protocol) and lost an average of 4 kg. For the 27 patients (79.4%) who lost weight, they experienced a decrease in symptoms by 75% compared with baseline using a modified DeMeester questionnaire.

Conversely, Kjellin and colleagues[69] randomized 20 obese patients with GERD to a very low-caloric diet (VLCD, approximately 800 Kcal/d) or no change in diet. Patients in the VLCD group lost an average of 10.8 kg, and the control group gained 0.6 kg. Those on the VLCD did not have significant changes in reflux symptoms. The control group was then given the VLCD and lost weight but again no change in symptoms were observed. Frederiksen and colleagues[70] studied 34 morbidly obese patients who were prescribed liquid VLCD pre- and post-vertical banded gastroplasty and found no change in acid exposure time from baseline compared with 10 to 14 days after the start of VLCD or 3 weeks after surgery.

Bariatric Surgery and GERD

The use of bariatric surgery has increased over the past 2 decades as it has proved to be an effective treatment of obesity. In 2006, the number of bariatric operations in the United States was reported as 112,999.[71] Bariatric surgeries can be classified as restrictive, malabsorptive, or both. In restrictive surgeries, the gastric anatomy is altered to reduce gastric volume to induce early satiety, which in turn leads to weight loss. Examples of restrictive surgeries include vertical banded gastroplasty, intragastric balloon, sleeve gastrectomy (SG) and laparoscopic adjustable gastric banding (LAGB). Malabsorptive surgeries induce malabsorption by shortening the gut, and/or altering the time food is subjected to digestive juices. Examples of malabsorptive surgeries include biliopancreatic diversion with and without duodenal switch and jejunoileal bypass. Combined techniques include Roux-en-Y gastric bypass (RYGB).

There have been several studies published that have examined changes in GERD symptoms after bariatric surgery. These studies have generally been prospective cohort and retrospective studies and not randomized controlled studies. Analysis of results is confounded by the common practice of repairing hiatal hernias during surgery and the heterogeneity in post-bariatric diet, lifestyle modification, and PPI use.

The most common bariatric surgeries performed are the RYGB, LAGB,[71] and more recently the SG.[72] RYGB involves stapling of the stomach to create a small ($\leq$30 mL) upper gastric pouch.[73] A roux limb of jejunum is then anastomosed to the gastric pouch bypassing absorptive surface area. Potential mechanism for RYGB reducing GERD symptoms include diverting bile away from the esophagus,[74] eliminating acid production in the gastric pouch,[75] or reducing volume of acid refluxate.[76] De Groot and colleagues[77] performed a systematic review on bariatric surgery and the effects on GERD. They identified 8 studies that evaluated GERD symptoms after RYGB and 3 studies that compared RYGB to other weight loss techniques with respect to GERD symptoms. All studies showed an improvement in GERD symptoms after RYGB except one by Korenkov and colleagues.[78] Most of the studies included in the systematic review used questionnaires (QUEST) and only 4 of the 11 studies used objective measurements (ie, endoscopy, 24-h pH monitoring) to define GERD.

In LAGB, a band device is placed around the fundus of the stomach immediately below the esophagogastric junction, and a subcutaneous reservoir is used to adjust the band size.[77] In the same systematic review by De Groot and colleagues,[77] the effects of LAGB on GERD were analyzed. Of 12 studies identified, 4 reported a positive effect on GERD, 2 studies found a positive effect so long as there was no pouch dilatation and/or a prior esophageal motility disorder was not present, 2 studies showed an increase in symptoms based on pH metry, manometry, and/or endoscopic findings, and 4 studies showed conflicting data in different domains of the diagnostic tests. Because of the conflicting data it is difficult to come to a conclusion on the effects of LAGB on GERD symptoms.

In SG the stomach is vertically divided reducing the volume to about 25% of the original size. In a recent systematic review by Chiu and colleagues,[72] which included 15 studies of SG, 4 found a post-operative increase in GERD prevalence, 7 showed reduced prevalence, and in 4 studies the prevalence before and after surgery could not be determined. As with most studies examining the effects of bariatric surgery on GERD, there was significant heterogeneity between studies including differences in follow-up time ranging from 6 months to 5 years, differences in the case definition of GERD, and lack of control groups. Therefore, similar to LAGB, it is difficult to come to conclusively determine the effects of SG on GERD.

In summary, surgical management is an effective approach to weight loss, and the data has generally shown that this weight loss can have positive effects on GERD. RYGB studies have provided the most consistent evidence for reducing GERD after surgery. Thus, in patients with severe GERD preoperatively, preferential consideration should be given to performing RYGB as the bariatric procedure of choice.

SUMMARY

Epidemiologic studies strongly suggest that the prevalence of GERD is increasing, and the major contributing factor to this trend is the rising prevalence of obesity. This trend has been observed in the United States as well as in Europe and Eastern Asia. Central obesity as opposed to BMI appears to be a better marker for the risks of metaplastic and neoplastic complications of GERD. Visceral adipose tissue secretes hormonal mediators, which may increase the risk of BE and esophageal adenocarcinoma. Studies have preliminarily shown that leptin levels have a direct relationship with the development of BE, and adiponectin levels are inversely related. Other factors that may play a role in the pathophysiology of GERD due to obesity include the increased prevalence of esophageal motor disorders, higher number of transient relaxations of the lower esophageal sphincter, and increased intra-abdominal pressure. The benefit of weight loss through diet as a means to decrease GERD symptoms is not yet established. However, gastric bypass surgery leads to substantial weight loss and the data have consistently shown a decrease in GERD symptoms. Unfortunately, only a few studies have included pH data to confirm improvement after surgery.

REFERENCES

1. Hom C, Vaezi MF. Extraesophageal manifestations of gastroesophageal reflux disease. Gastroenterol Clin North Am 2013;42(1):71–91.
2. El-Serag HB, Sweet S, Winchester CC, et al. Update on the epidemiology of gastro-oesophageal reflux disease: a systematic review. Gut 2013. [Epub ahead of print].
3. El-Serag H. The association between obesity and GERD: a review of the epidemiological evidence. Dig Dis Sci 2008;53(9):2307–12.
4. El-Serag HB, Hashmi A, Garcia J, et al. Visceral abdominal obesity measured by CT scan is associated with an increased risk of Barrett's oesophagus: a case-control study. Gut 2013. [Epub ahead of print].
5. Flegal KM, Carroll MD, Kit BK, et al. Prevalence of obesity and trends in the distribution of body mass index among US adults, 1999-2010. JAMA 2012;307(5):491–7.
6. Jacobson BC, Somers SC, Fuchs CS, et al. Body-mass index and symptoms of gastroesophageal reflux in women. N Engl J Med 2006;354(22):2340–8.
7. Corley DA, Kubo A, Zhao W. Abdominal obesity, ethnicity and gastro-oesophageal reflux symptoms. Gut 2007;56(6):756–62.
8. El-Serag HB, Graham DY, Satia JA, et al. Obesity is an independent risk factor for GERD symptoms and erosive esophagitis. Am J Gastroenterol 2005;100(6):1243–50.
9. Cremonini F, Locke GR 3rd, Schleck CD, et al. Relationship between upper gastrointestinal symptoms and changes in body weight in a population-based cohort. Neurogastroenterol Motil 2006;18(11):987–94.
10. Nandurkar S, Locke GR 3rd, Fett S, et al. Relationship between body mass index, diet, exercise and gastro-oesophageal reflux symptoms in a community. Aliment Pharmacol Ther 2004;20(5):497–505.
11. von Ruesten A, Steffen A, Floegel A, et al. Trend in obesity prevalence in European adult cohort populations during follow-up since 1996 and their predictions to 2015. PLoS One 2011;6(11):e27455.
12. Nocon M, Labenz J, Willich SN. Lifestyle factors and symptoms of gastro-oesophageal reflux – a population-based study. Aliment Pharmacol Ther 2006;23(1):169–74.

13. Murray L, Johnston B, Lane A, et al. Relationship between body mass and gastro-oesophageal reflux symptoms: the Bristol Helicobacter Project. Int J Epidemiol 2003;32(4):645–50.

14. Diaz-Rubio M, Moreno-Elola-Olaso C, Rey E, et al. Symptoms of gastro-oesophageal reflux: prevalence, severity, duration and associated factors in a Spanish population. Aliment Pharmacol Ther 2004;19(1):95–105.

15. Rey E, Moreno-Elola-Olaso C, Artalejo FR, et al. Association between weight gain and symptoms of gastroesophageal reflux in the general population. Am J Gastroenterol 2006;101(2):229–33.

16. Nilsson M, Johnsen R, Ye W, et al. Obesity and estrogen as risk factors for gastroesophageal reflux symptoms. JAMA 2003;290(1):66–72.

17. Kang MS, Park DI, Oh SY, et al. Abdominal obesity is an independent risk factor for erosive esophagitis in a Korean population. J Gastroenterol Hepatol 2007; 22(10):1656–61.

18. Ma XQ, Cao Y, Wang R, et al. Prevalence of, and factors associated with, gastro-esophageal reflux disease: a population-based study in Shanghai, China. Dis Esophagus 2009;22(4):317–22.

19. Lagergren J, Bergstrom R, Nyren O. No relation between body mass and gastro-oesophageal reflux symptoms in a Swedish population based study. Gut 2000;47(1):26–9.

20. Martinez JA, Moreno B, Martinez-Gonzalez MA. Prevalence of obesity in Spain. Obes Rev 2004;5(3):171–2.

21. Ponce J, Vegazo O, Beltran B, et al. Prevalence of gastro-oesophageal reflux disease in Spain and associated factors. Aliment Pharmacol Ther 2006;23(1): 175–84.

22. Thorburn AW. Prevalence of obesity in Australia. Obes Rev 2005;6(3):187–9.

23. Moraes-Filho JP, Chinzon D, Eisig JN, et al. Prevalence of heartburn and gastro-esophageal reflux disease in the urban Brazilian population. Arq Gastroenterol 2005;42(2):122–7.

24. Rtveladze K, Marsh T, Webber L, et al. Health and economic burden of obesity in Brazil. PLoS One 2013;8(7):e68785.

25. He J, Ma X, Zhao Y, et al. A population-based survey of the epidemiology of symptom-defined gastroesophageal reflux disease: the Systematic Investigation of Gastrointestinal Diseases in China. BMC Gastroenterol 2010;10:94.

26. Wang Y, Mi J, Shan XY, et al. Is China facing an obesity epidemic and the consequences? The trends in obesity and chronic disease in China. Int J Obes (Lond) 2007;31(1):177–88.

27. Bhatia SJ, Reddy DN, Ghoshal UC, et al. Epidemiology and symptom profile of gastroesophageal reflux in the Indian population: report of the Indian Society of Gastroenterology Task Force. Indian J Gastroenterol 2011;30(3):118–27.

28. Griffiths PL, Bentley ME. The nutrition transition is underway in India. J Nutr 2001;131(10):2692–700.

29. Lee HL, Eun CS, Lee OY, et al. Association between GERD-related erosive esophagitis and obesity. J Clin Gastroenterol 2008;42(6):672–5.

30. Hampel H, Abraham NS, El-Serag HB. Meta-analysis: obesity and the risk for gastroesophageal reflux disease and its complications. Ann Intern Med 2005; 143(3):199–211.

31. Stein DJ, El-Serag HB, Kuczynski J, et al. The association of body mass index with Barrett's oesophagus. Aliment Pharmacol Ther 2005;22(10):1005–10.

32. Corley DA, Kubo A, Levin TR, et al. Abdominal obesity and body mass index as risk factors for Barrett's esophagus. Gastroenterology 2007;133(1):34–41 [quiz: 311].

33. Edelstein ZR, Bronner MP, Rosen SN, et al. Risk factors for Barrett's esophagus among patients with gastroesophageal reflux disease: a community clinic-based case-control study. Am J Gastroenterol 2009;104(4):834–42.

34. Rubenstein JH, Morgenstern H, Chey WD, et al. Protective role of gluteofemoral obesity in erosive oesophagitis and Barrett's oesophagus. Gut 2013. [Epub ahead of print].

35. Smith KJ, O'Brien SM, Smithers BM, et al. Interactions among smoking, obesity, and symptoms of acid reflux in Barrett's esophagus. Cancer Epidemiol Biomarkers Prev 2005;14(11 Pt 1):2481–6.

36. Veugelers PJ, Porter GA, Guernsey DL, et al. Obesity and lifestyle risk factors for gastroesophageal reflux disease, Barrett esophagus and esophageal adeno-carcinoma. Dis Esophagus 2006;19(5):321–8.

37. Pohl H, Welch HG. The role of overdiagnosis and reclassification in the marked increase of esophageal adenocarcinoma incidence. J Natl Cancer Inst 2005; 97(2):142–6.

38. Chow WH, Blot WJ, Vaughan TL, et al. Body mass index and risk of adenocar-cinomas of the esophagus and gastric cardia. J Natl Cancer Inst 1998;90(2): 150–5.

39. Hoyo C, Cook MB, Kamangar F, et al. Body mass index in relation to oeso-phageal and oesophagogastric junction adenocarcinomas: a pooled analysis from the International BEACON Consortium. Int J Epidemiol 2012;41(6): 1706–18.

40. Engel LS, Chow WH, Vaughan TL, et al. Population attributable risks of esoph-ageal and gastric cancers. J Natl Cancer Inst 2003;95(18):1404–13.

41. Suter M, Dorta G, Giusti V, et al. Gastro-esophageal reflux and esophageal motility disorders in morbidly obese patients. Obes Surg 2004;14(7):959–66.

42. Koppman JS, Poggi L, Szomstein S, et al. Esophageal motility disorders in the morbidly obese population. Surg Endosc 2007;21(5):761–4.

43. Jaffin BW, Knoepflmacher P, Greenstein R. High prevalence of asymptomatic esophageal motility disorders among morbidly obese patients. Obes Surg 1999;9(4):390–5.

44. Hong D, Khajanchee YS, Pereira N, et al. Manometric abnormalities and gastro-esophageal reflux disease in the morbidly obese. Obes Surg 2004;14:744–9.

45. Quiroga E, Cuenca-Abente F, Flum D, et al. Impaired esophageal function in morbidly obese patients with gastroesophageal reflux disease: evaluation with multichannel intraluminal impedance. Surg Endosc 2006;20(5):739–43.

46. Kouklakis G, Moschos J, Kountouras J, et al. Relationship between obesity and gastroesophageal reflux disease as recorded by 3-hour esophageal pH moni-toring. Rom J Gastroenterol 2005;14(2):117–21.

47. Kahrilas PJ, Shi G, Manka M, et al. Increased frequency of transient lower esophageal sphincter relaxation induced by gastric distention in reflux patients with hiatal hernia. Gastroenterology 2000;118(4):688–95.

48. Fisher BL, Pennathur A, Mutnick JL, et al. Obesity correlates with gastroesoph-ageal reflux. Dig Dis Sci 1999;44(11):2290–4.

49. Wu JC, Mui LM, Cheung CM, et al. Obesity is associated with increased tran-sient lower esophageal sphincter relaxation. Gastroenterology 2007;132(3): 883–9.

50. Pandolfino JE, El-Serag HB, Zhang Q, et al. Obesity: a challenge to esophago-gastric junction integrity. Gastroenterology 2006;130(3):639–49.

51. Lambert DM, Marceau S, Forse RA. Intra-abdominal pressure in the morbidly obese. Obes Surg 2005;15(9):1225–32.

52. Varela JE, Hinojosa M, Nguyen N. Correlations between intra-abdominal pressure and obesity-related co-morbidities. Surg Obes Relat Dis 2009;5(5):524–8.

53. El-Serag HB, Tran T, Richardson P, et al. Anthropometric correlates of intragastric pressure. Scand J Gastroenterol 2006;41(8):887–91.

54. Geliebter A, Hashim SA. Gastric capacity in normal, obese, and bulimic women. Physiol Behav 2001;74(4–5):743–6.

55. Granstrom L, Backman L. Stomach distension in extremely obese and in normal subjects. Acta Chir Scand 1985;151(4):367–70.

56. Zahorska-Markiewicz B, Jonderko K, Lelek A, et al. Gastric emptying and obesity. Hum Nutr Clin Nutr 1986;40(4):309–13.

57. Wright RA, Krinksy S, Fleeman C, et al. Gastric emptying and obesity. Gastroenterology 1983;84(4):747–51.

58. Tosetti C, Corinaldesi R, Stangellini V, et al. Gastric emptying of solids in morbid obesity. Int J Obes Relat Metab Disord 1996;20(3):200–5.

59. Buchholz V, Berkenstadt H, Goitein D, et al. Gastric emptying is not prolonged in obese patients. Surg Obes Relat Dis 2013;9(5):714–7.

60. Kelesidis I, Kelesidis T, Mantzoros CS. Adiponectin and cancer: a systematic review. Br J Cancer 2006;94(9):1221–5.

61. Rubenstein JH, Dahlkemper A, Kao JY, et al. A pilot study of the association of low plasma adiponectin and Barrett's esophagus. Am J Gastroenterol 2008; 103(6):1358–64.

62. Rubenstein JH, Kao JY, Madanick RD, et al. Association of adiponectin multimers with Barrett's oesophagus. Gut 2009;58(12):1583–9.

63. Weigle DS. Leptin and other secretory products of adipocytes modulate multiple physiological functions. Ann Endocrinol (Paris) 1997;58(2):132–6.

64. Ogunwobi O, Mutungi G, Beales IL. Leptin stimulates proliferation and inhibits apoptosis in Barrett's esophageal adenocarcinoma cells by cyclooxygenase-2-dependent, prostaglandin-E2-mediated transactivation of the epidermal growth factor receptor and c-Jun NH2-terminal kinase activation. Endocrinology 2006;147(9):4505–16.

65. Kendall BJ, Macdonald GA, Hayward NK, et al. Leptin and the risk of Barrett's oesophagus. Gut 2008;57(4):448–54.

66. Ness-Jensen E, Lindam A, Lagergren J, et al. Weight loss and reduction in gastroesophageal reflux. A prospective population-based cohort study: the HUNT study. Am J Gastroenterol 2013;108(3):376–82.

67. Singh M, Lee J, Gupta N, et al. Weight loss can lead to resolution of gastroesophageal reflux disease symptoms: a prospective intervention trial. Obesity (Silver Spring) 2013;21(2):284–90.

68. Fraser-Moodie CA, Norton B, Gornall C, et al. Weight loss has an independent beneficial effect on symptoms of gastro-oesophageal reflux in patients who are overweight. Scand J Gastroenterol 1999;34(4):337–40.

69. Kjellin A, Ramel S, Rossner S, et al. Gastroesophageal reflux in obese patients is not reduced by weight reduction. Scand J Gastroenterol 1996; 31(11):1047–51.

70. Frederiksen SG, Johansson J, Johnsson F, et al. Neither low-calorie diet nor vertical banded gastroplasty influence gastro-oesophageal reflux in morbidly obese patients. Eur J Surg 2000;166(4):296–300.

71. Livingston EH. The incidence of bariatric surgery has plateaued in the U.S. Am J Surg 2010;200(3):378–85.

72. Chiu S, Birch DW, Shi X, et al. Effect of sleeve gastrectomy on gastroesophageal reflux disease: a systematic review. Surg Obes Relat Dis 2011;7(4):510–5.

73. DeMaria EJ. Bariatric surgery for morbid obesity. N Engl J Med 2007;356(21): 2176–83.
74. Frezza EE, Ikramuddin S, Gourash W, et al. Symptomatic improvement in gastroesophageal reflux disease (GERD) following laparoscopic Roux-en-Y gastric bypass. Surg Endosc 2002;16(7):1027–31.
75. Cobey F, Oelschlager B. Complete regression of Barrett's esophagus after Roux-en-Y gastric bypass. Obes Surg 2005;15(5):710–2.
76. Smith SC, Edwards CB, Goodman GN. Symptomatic and clinical improvement in morbidly obese patients with gastroesophageal reflux disease following Roux-en-Y gastric bypass. Obes Surg 1997;7(6):479–84.
77. De Groot NL, Burgerhart JS, Van De Meeberg PC, et al. Systematic review: the effects of conservative and surgical treatment for obesity on gastro-oesophageal reflux disease. Aliment Pharmacol Ther 2009;30(11–12):1091–102.
78. Korenkov M, Kohler L, Yucel N, et al. Esophageal motility and reflux symptoms before and after bariatric surgery. Obes Surg 2002;12(1):72–6.

Index

Note: Page numbers of article titles are in **boldface** type.

Gastroenterol Clin N Am 43 (2014) 175–183
http://dx.doi.org/10.1016/S0889-8553(14)00010-7
0889-8553/14/$ – see front matter © 2014 Elsevier Inc. All rights reserved.

gastro.theclinics.com

Moving?

Make sure your subscription moves with you!

To notify us of your new address, find your **Clinics Account Number** (located on your mailing label above your name), and contact customer service at:

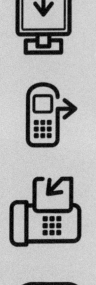

Email: journalscustomerservice-usa@elsevier.com

800-654-2452 (subscribers in the U.S. & Canada)
314-447-8871 (subscribers outside of the U.S. & Canada)

Fax number: 314-447-8029

Elsevier Health Sciences Division
Subscription Customer Service
3251 Riverport Lane
Maryland Heights, MO 63043

*To ensure uninterrupted delivery of your subscription, please notify us at least 4 weeks in advance of move.

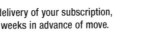

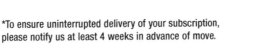

Printed and bound by CPI Group (UK) Ltd, Croydon, CR0 4YY

03/10/2024

01040496-0018